This book is dedicated to all of our patients who allowed us to care for them and restore their hopes and their dreams.

100 Questions & Answers About Head and Neck Cancer

Elise Carper, RN, MA, APRN, BC, AOCN

Director of Nursing and Adult Nurse Practitioner
Department of Radiation Oncology
Continuum Cancer Centers of New York
New York City

Kenneth Hu, MD

Attending Radiation Oncologist
Department of Radiation Oncology
Continuum Cancer Centers of New York
New York City

Elena Kuzin, RN, MSN, APRN, BC, AOCN

Geriatric and Adult Nurse Practitioner
Department of Radiation Oncology
Continuum Cancer Centers of New York
New York City

JONES AND BARTLETT PUBLISHERS

Sudbury, Massachusetts

BOSTON   TORONTO   LONDON   SINGAPORE

World Headquarters

Jones and Bartlett Publishers
40 Tall Pine Drive
Sudbury, MA 01776
978-443-5000
info@jbpub.com
www.jbpub.com

Jones and Bartlett Publishers
Canada
6339 Ormindale Way
Mississauga, Ontario L5V 1J2
CANADA

Jones and Bartlett Publishers
International
Barb House, Barb Mews
London W6 7PA
UK

Jones and Bartlett's books and products are available through most bookstores and online booksellers. To contact Jones and Bartlett Publishers directly, call 800-832-0034, fax 978-443-8000, or visit our Web site, www.jbpub.com.

Substantial discounts on bulk quantities of Jones and Bartlett's publications are available to corporations, professional associations, and other qualified organizations. For details and specific discount information, contact the special sales department at Jones and Bartlett via the above contact information or send an email to specialsales@jbpub.com.

The authors, editor, and publisher have made every effort to provide accurate information. However, they are not responsible for errors, omissions, or for any outcomes related to the use of the contents of this book and take no responsibility for the use of the products and procedures described. Treatments and side effects described in this book may not be applicable to all people; likewise, some people may require a dose or experience a side effect that is not described herein. Drugs and medical devices are discussed that may have limited availability controlled by the Food and Drug Administration (FDA) for use only in a research study or clinical trial. Research, clinical practice, and government regulations often change the accepted standard in this field. When consideration is being given to use of any drug in the clinical setting, the health care provider or reader is responsible for determining FDA status of the drug, reading the package insert, and reviewing prescribing information for the most up-to-date recommendations on dose, precautions, and contraindications, and determining the appropriate usage for the product. This is especially important in the case of drugs that are new or seldom used.

Production Credits

Executive Publisher: Christopher Davis
Associate Editor: Kathy Richardson
Production Director: Amy Rose
Production Assistant: Mike Boblitt
Manufacturing Buyer: Therese Connell
Composition: Appingo

Cover Design: Jonathan Ayotte
Cover Image: Woman with head in hand ©
    Photodisc; man © Photodisc; woman with
    cup © Radu Razvan/ShutterStock, Inc.
Printing and Binding: Malloy, Inc.
Cover Printing: Malloy, Inc.

Library of Congress Cataloging-in-Publication Data
Carper, Elise.
    100 questions and answers about head and neck cancer / Elise Carper, Kenneth Hu, and Elena Kuzin.
        p. cm.
    Includes index.
    ISBN-13: 978-0-7637-4307-9
    ISBN-10: 0-7637-4307-0
    1. Head--Cancer--Miscellanea. 2. Neck--Cancer--Miscellanea. I. Hu, Kenneth. II. Kuzin, Elena. III. Title. IV. Title: One hundred questions and answers about head and neck cancer.
    RC280.H4C372 2008
    616.99'491--dc22
                                2007017092
6048

Printed in the United States of America
11 10 09 08 07   10 9 8 7 6 5 4 3 2 1

CONTENTS

Until I was diagnosed with cancer on the floor of my mouth, I had never heard of head and neck cancer. I did not know of anyone who had such a cancer, nor did I know that there were physicians who specialized in the treatment of this kind of cancer. When I was diagnosed in 1990, I had no computer to research my disease, nor were there resources in the libraries. Medical books explaining head and neck cancer were too complex for the layperson to understand, and there were no support groups to provide information and support for head and neck cancer survivors.

My sources of information were limited. I had the 1-800 4-Cancer number that I could call for information and a brochure from the National Cancer Institute, entitled, "Oral Cancer." My surgeon was more than willing to answer any questions that I had, but therein lay the problem. I didn't know what questions to ask. In my mind, I had a tumor. The surgeon would remove it, and life would go on as it had before. It was that simple! But it wasn't that simple! No one can be completely prepared for what lies ahead after receiving a diagnosis of cancer, and I certainly didn't know a lot about head and neck cancer.

So just what is head and neck cancer? For the majority of people this question has little meaning, but for those of us who have been diagnosed with this disease, it is a question that has many answers, most of which we only come to understand during our cancer journey.

That initial discussion with the doctor when the diagnosis is given leaves the patient overwhelmed, frightened, and yet needing to know all about the cancer but not knowing what questions to ask. *100 Questions & Answers About Head and Neck Cancer*, written in lay language, is a resource for the newly diagnosed patient and family member who is not familiar with this type of cancer. This book presents the questions that need to be asked with the answers that help to educate the patient and family about the disease.

Through the questions and answers found in this book, the patient becomes more aware of his/her disease, the treatment, the options that are available, the support and encouragement that can be had, as well as other resources that may help the individual to cope with the many aspects of head and neck cancer. Commentary by head and neck cancer survivors helps the reader to see the situations through the eyes of one who has successfully been treated for the disease and who has moved on with his/her life.

Times have changed considerably in the past 17 years since I was diagnosed. With the help of the Internet, oral and head and neck cancer patients now have an abundance of information at their fingertips in addition to new books and brochures about their disease. Moreover, Support for People with Oral and Head and Neck Cancer (SPOHNC), an organization dedicated to raising awareness and meeting the needs of oral and head and neck cancer patients, now has chapters of its organization offering support and information throughout the United States.

Nancy E. Leupold
President and Founder
SPOHNC

In the summer of 2002, the word cancer seemed like a misprint to me: To that first letter 'c'—an asymmetrical backwards crescent moon—add a vertical slash reaching ecstatically from earth to sky to get a 'd.' I was a vibrant young dancer touring the world as a performer and teacher, never smoked in my life, and my feet firmly planted in the belief of myself as invincible, young, strong, and healthy. I was a powerful modern dancer, rythmic and muscular, not the delicate and fragile sylph ballerina that I moved to New York City at age 16 to become. But, in 2002, I would be back in NYC, in the Union Square and Lincoln Center neighborhoods only blocks from the buildings where I had forged a professional dance career, delicate and fragile as a sylph—a bald and hungry insect, not a chiffon winged ballerina.

At the moment of diagnosis, the firm ground upon which my self-image was confidently planted immediately disintegrated, leaving me paddling as I was instantly tossed into waves of unknowns. This ocean had no solid edge, no clean finish, no absolute neatness of assurance that I would be back to my old life, feeling great, on exactly this date and time. Gasping for air, there may have been brief waves of shock and fear, but I let those pass quickly, to be replaced with questions. For every answer and for every unanswerable, I echoed back with hope, for that is what I felt I needed the most, in order to flow through this unfathomable change. All that I had clung to fell away, like skins of outgrown personas, in this vast primordial ocean of survival, and I molted into a thin spirit of pure intuition and positive belief in the power of life force itself.

This ocean imagery became even more visible, after I was fitted for my tight plastic net of a radiation mask, which left me with indented pattern on my face, like the fins and scales of a mermaid on the streets of Union Square!

The letter W looks like a wave, and indeed it is found in Who What Where When Why how, which I assembled in every possible combination. What was next, when would treatments start/begin, how long would this last, what side effects, were there experimental medicines being considered, where would I have treatments, who would be by my side, how would their lives be affected, how could this have happened, when could I go back to dancing…?

I found it important to not passively expect that I would be told what to do, to wait for 'snap,' a magic cure button. I wanted to understand what was happening to my body, to the fine instrument I had so trusted and relied upon. I wanted to be an active creative collaborator in my healing and recovery, as I was in all the choreographies that life had presented to me thus far. I certainly encourage all cancer patients to have the courage to find out as much as they can from every resource available to them, from research and reading, to questions for doctors, to trading anecdotes in the hospital waiting room with other patients about what one might expect and how to alleviate discomfort. (Continued thanks to Tom and Caroline Law who let me know, among other things, that the aloe vera gel and juice would indeed help with the radiation symptoms!)

Hence, many, many, many questions emerged from me, from simple to complex, inquisitive about past, present, and future. What is self-explanatory about cancer when you are surviving it? Nothing; I took nothing for granted. Even in the radiation waiting room, I noticed that other patients were curious about the yoga and breathing I was doing to relax, and I was so happy to respond to their questions by showing them simple exercises, and even more delighted when they quickly experienced positive results. (I call it, "Breath of Life"!)

Dr. Hu was absolutely thorough and caring in his response to every one of my questions; he was updated on the most obscure articles I had come across, and learned the names and personal details of the constantly changing assortment of family members, friends, and colleagues who accompanied me to my daily radiation sessions. Indeed I felt like I was his only patient! He certainly embodies the true healer, not only a doctor, as does his caring staff of nurses and radiation team. Another truly helpful aspect was that because of the Continuum protocol program, he worked in direct coordination with my brilliant and compassionate surgeon Dr. Peter Costantino and the kind chemotherapy doctor and marathon runner Dr. Culliney. I don't think it can be easy for these doctors to face so many patients day after day, each one struggling to face one of the greatest fears of modern civilization, but these men and their office staff, interns, and nurses stand out as truly extraordinary human beings, knowledgeability hand in hand with true caring. The light of their collective spirit was radiant in this dark and challenging time of change.

Even now, almost four years after the finish of treatment (and still a year away from being pronounced 'cured') I still go to my 3–6 months exams with my doctors and have many questions, about the latest findings I have read about possible causes for this kind of cancer, about various complementary protocols I am trying, and new treatments being tested. I am slowly returning to performing, teaching, and have become a choreographer, even an actress, working in two major films since my cancer diagnosis. People can't believe I was ever sick, and although I am aware of many subtle changes, I am only grateful for the medicines (surgery, chemo, radiation, and other complementary therapies and spiritual practices), which have contributed to me being able to live fully and share with the earth all the qualities that are my uniquely special offerings. Indeed, a week doesn't go by in which I can dwell on anything but loving gratitude, for I am constantly being contacted by friends who have loved ones who have been diagnosed with cancer, and they are seeking out hope, guidance, and direction for their own oceans of unknowns. I feel honored to now be able to recommend this book, which will be an invaluable resource for others who are stepping into this passage of change.

With a dancing spirit,
Rulan Tangen

A diagnosis of head and neck cancer is a frightening experience for any patient. Beyond the usual fears about life and death, there are the added concerns about form and function. Such vital capabilities as speech, swallowing, vision, and taste can be profoundly affected by the cancer and its treatment. Additional concerns about appearance and social interaction may also arise. To make matters even more complex, there are often multiple treatment options, combination and sequences of treatment, all of which have side effects, complications, risks, and benefits. Thus, perhaps more than any other group of cancer patients, head and neck cancer patients have many questions and need comprehensive answers.

This book, *100 Question & Answers About Head and Neck Cancer*, by Elise Carper, Kenneth Hu, and Elena Kuzin, fulfills this important need. The authors are enormously experienced in the management of these diseases, literally having treated thousands of patients. They have compiled their rich experience and expertise in a readable, simple format. There is no doubt that countless patients with tumors of the head and neck, as well as their loved ones and caregivers, will find answers and comfort in these pages.

Louis B. Harrison, MD

Clinical Director, Continuum Cancer Centers of New York

Chairman of Radiation Oncology, Beth Israel Medical Center and St. Luke's-Roosevelt Hospital

Professor of Radiation Oncology, Albert Einstein College of Medicine

Co-Director, Institute for Head, Neck, and Thyroid Cancer

PART ONE

The Basics

What is cancer?

Is cancer a tumor?

How does the pathologist get the cells?

More . . .

Cancer

a term used to describe diseases caused by abnormal cell growth and behavior

Metastasis

the multiplication and spreading of cancer cells to other parts of the body

Tumor

a term used to describe a mass or lump in the body

Malignant

a tumor composed of cancer cells

Benign

a tumor composed of non-cancerous cells

Pathologist

a doctor trained to look at tumor cells under a microscope to determine whether they are benign or malignant

Grade

describes the aggressiveness of the tumor cells

Histology

where in the body the cells originate from

Biopsy

a procedure performed to obtain cells from the tumor to examine.

1. What is cancer?

The term **cancer** is used to describe diseases caused by abnormal cell growth and behavior. There are over 100 different diseases called cancer, each usually named for the type of cell or organ it originated from. Regardless of where the cancer may spread it is always named for the place where it started. For example, abnormal cells arising from tongue tissue are called tongue cancer cells. All the cells of the body multiply and divide but stop multiplying when the body no longer needs them. The structure and behavior of cancer cells is somehow changed and cancer cells multiply and divide uncontrollably. These cells then spread, invading and injuring normal tissues and breaking off and traveling to other organs of the body. This is called **metastasis**.

2. Is cancer a tumor?

The term **tumor** is used to describe a lump or mass found in the body. A tumor composed of cancer cells is called **malignant**. A **benign** tumor does not spread to other parts of the body and, with very rare exceptions, is not life-threatening. To determine if a tumor is benign or malignant, the cells of the mass must be examined under a microscope. A specially trained doctor (a **pathologist**) looks at the tumor cells and determines if the cells are cancerous or not. The pathologist also determines how aggressive the cancer cells are (the **grade**), and from what body part the cells originated (the **histology**).

3. How does the pathologist get the cells?

Obtaining tumor cells to examine under a microscope is often done with a **biopsy**. Biopsies can be done by using a needle to remove a few cells from the tumor (a **fine needle aspiration**, or FNA). Sometimes a larger amount of tissue is needed and removal of a part of the tumor (incisional biopsy) or the entire tumor (excisional biopsy) is done.

Identifying the tumor histology and grade is one part of a process called **staging**. Staging refers to tests and examinations done to help determine the extent of the disease process, and whether the cancer has spread to other parts of the body. A thorough physical examination that may reveal swollen **lymph nodes** is part of staging. Radiologic and laboratory tests also help determine stage. Most cancers are divided into four stages. Stage I, the earliest stage, is the most limited, meaning the cancer is still within the tissue of origin. In Stage II, lymph nodes nearby have cancer cells within them. In Stage III the cancer has spread into surrounding tissues, and in Stage IV the cancer has spread to a distant part or organ of the body.

4. What makes a cell become a cancer cell?

Normal body cells grow, divide, and die in an orderly fashion. Normal cells divide rapidly in the early years of a person's life, until the person becomes an adult. After that, cells in most parts of the body divide only to replace worn-out or dying cells and to repair injuries.

Cancer is a condition where some cells fail to follow their cycle rules. Cancer cells develop because of damage to DNA. This substance is in every cell and directs all its activities. Most of the time when DNA becomes damaged, the body is able to repair it. In cancer cells, the damaged DNA is not repaired. People can inherit damaged DNA, which accounts for inherited cancers. Often, though, a person's DNA becomes damaged by exposure to something in the environment, like smoking.

Cancer usually develops as a tumor. Some cancers, like leukemia, do not form tumors. Instead, leukemia cells involve the blood and blood-forming organs and circulate through other tissues where they grow.

Different types of cancer can behave very differently. For example, tonsil cancer and lung cancer are very different dis-

The Basics

Fine Needle Aspiration (FNA)
the insertion of a small bore needle (a needle with a small diameter) into a tumor and then the removal (aspiration) of cells

Staging
the tests or examinations done to help determine the extent of the disease process. This also determines whether or not the tumor has spread to other parts of the body.

Lymph Nodes
small, round, oval or bean-shaped structures that filter lymph fluid of unwanted materials such as bacteria and cancer cells

Staging refers to tests and examinations done to help determine the extent of the disease process, and whether the cancer has spread to other parts of the body.

eases. They grow at different rates and respond to different treatments. This is why people with cancer need treatment that is aimed at their specific cancer.

5. Are all cancers of the head and neck the same?

The term "head and neck" refers to many separate and different organs of the body, all found above the shoulders, excluding the brain and spinal cord. Cancers within the head and neck likewise are completely unique and separate from each other. For example, cancer of the lip is different from cancer of the tongue or voice box. The cells of lip cancer look different under the microscope from cells from tonsil cancer. The staging criteria—that is, what features make a specific tumor Stage II or Stage III—differ for a voice box tumor and a tumor of the cheek. Treatment for each of these cancers may be similar to one another or very different.

Many different cancers are included in the grouping termed "head and neck." Some are named for the organ they arise from such as lip, tongue, or nasal sinus cancers. Others are named for the area of the **pharynx** they arise from; **nasopharynx, hypopharynx, oropharynx,** and so on. The term pharynx is used to describe the airway space starting behind the nose, extending downward to the voice box and including the space within the mouth.

6. What is the nasopharynx? Where is it located?

The nasopharynx is the area behind the nose and between the eyes. It includes the airspace found there, as well as the lining of the walls, ceiling, and floor of the cavity. Tumors of the nasopharynx start to grow from the side wall of the space, and eventually fill the space. All of this mass is considered part of the nasopharynx tumor.

Pharynx
throat

Nasopharynx
the area behind the nose and between the eyes

Hypopharynx
includes the tissues of the lowest part of the throat, down to the level of the voice box (larynx)

Oropharynx
contains the soft palate, the uvula, the tonsils, the base of the tongue, and the wall of the pharynx (throat) from the soft palate to above the voice box

Many different cancers are included in the grouping termed "head and neck."

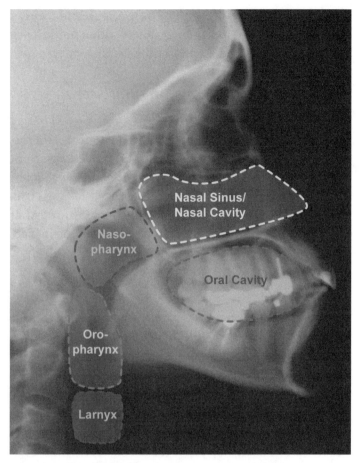

The Basics

Figure 1   Courtesy of Beth Israel Medical Center, New York, NY.

7. What are the nasal sinuses? Where are they found? How do they function?

The nasal sinuses are a complex group of air sacs found within the face (see Figure 1). The **maxillary sinuses** are spaces found in the cheeks, right above the maxilla or top jawbone. The **ethmoid sinus** is found between the eyebrows, behind the ethmoid bone. The **sphenoid sinuses** are found behind the sphenoid bone.

Maxillary Sinuses

spaces found in the cheeks, right above the maxilla

Ethmoid Sinus

found between the eyebrows

Sphenoid Sinuses

includes the tissues of the lowest part of the throat, down to the level of the voice box (larynx)

Sinuses are normally filled with air. When congested they can cause discomfort and pain. Tumors found within sinuses push against the walls of the airspace and cause discomfort.

8. What structures are found in the oral cavity? How do they function?

The oral cavity includes the lips, **gingiva** (or gums), **hard palate** (or roof of the mouth), **buccal mucosa** (or cheeks), tongue, floor of the mouth, and the **retromolar trigone**, which refers to the inside angle of the jaws. The lips bring in and then hold food within the mouth. The floor of the mouth and roof of the mouth, along with the cheeks, help hold the food in place so the tongue can move the food gradually to the back of the mouth to be swallowed.

9. What structures are found in the oropharynx? How do they function?

The oropharynx contains the **soft palate** (the soft part of the back of the roof of the mouth), the **uvula** (an extension of the soft palate that hangs down from the back of the roof of the mouth), the **tonsils** (soft lymphoid tissue on either side of the throat), the **base of the tongue** (the part of the tongue you can not see that extends down the throat to the voice box), and the wall of the pharynx (throat) from the soft palate to above the voice box. The soft palate helps prevent food from going up into the nasopharynx and out the nose. The tonsils are lymphoid tissue that may assist the immune system of the body to fight infection. The base of the tongue works with the oral part of the tongue to move food from the mouth down to the stomach.

10. What structures are found in the hypopharynx? How do they function?

The hypopharynx includes the tissues of the lowest part of the throat, down to the level of the voice box, or **larynx**. The

Gingiva

gums in the mouth

Hard Palate

the roof of the mouth

Buccal Mucosa

cheeks

Retromolar Trigone

inside angle of the jaws

Soft Palate

the soft part of the back of the roof of the mouth

Uvula

an extension of the soft palate that hangs down from the back of the roof of the mouth

Tonsils

soft lymphoid tissue on both sides of the throat

Base of the Tongue

the part of the tongue you can not see that extends down the throat to the voice box

Larynx

the voice box

pyriform sinuses are air spaces on either side of the voice box. The walls of the throat or pharynx, at the level of the voice box, moving downward to the top of the esophagus, are also included in this subcategory. This part of the throat connects the mouth with the esophagus.

Pyriform Sinuses
air spaces on either side of the voice box (larynx)

The Basics

11. What is the larynx? How does it function?

The larynx, or "voice box," is actually made up of several different organs. The vocal cords are two small organs on either side of the voice box that move together and apart to create sound. These organs are connected by cartilage to the sides of the voice box. Above the vocal cords is the area of the larynx called the supraglottic larynx. The epiglottis is a flap of tissue that closes over the voice box during swallowing. The swallowing movement prevents food from entering the lungs.

12. What are lymph nodes?

Lymph nodes are small, round, oval, or bean-shaped structures found along lymphatic vessels throughout the body. They filter lymph fluid of unwanted materials such as bacteria and cancer cells before it returns the lymph to the blood. At times of infection or injury, lymph nodes swell as they work to cleanse the lymph, shrinking back to normal after the infection clears or the injury heals.

13. What does it mean if the cancer has spread to the lymph nodes?

Cancer cells often spread through lymph channels to lymph nodes. Swollen lymph nodes are commonly seen in cancers of the head and neck. Cancers sometimes start in organs of the head and neck, like the nasopharynx, but are undetectable. When the cancer cells spread to the lymph nodes of the neck, the nodes will swell, and this often leads to the diagnosis of cancer.

Computerized Axial Tomography (CAT) scans

a computed axial tomography scan is often used to evaluate the anatomical regions of the head and neck and to locate abnormalities

Positron Emission Tomography (PET) scans

shows the functional status of your body, by evaluating cell metabolism. It images areas of the body where high rates of glucose metabolism exist.

Involvement of the lymph nodes is the single most important predictor of how likely a cancer is to be cured.

Involvement of the lymph nodes is the single most important predictor of how likely a cancer is to be cured. If just a single lymph node is found to have cancer spread, the chance of being cured is decreased by up to 50%. **Computerized Axial Tomography (CAT) scans, Positron Emission Tomography (PET) scans, MRI, and physical examination are the best way to assess lymph node involvement.**

Lymph node spread. If your biopsy comes back negative, have it taken out anyway. These biopsies are often false negative.

- Rob Jaffe, patient

14. Are all cancers of the head and neck fatal?

No. Cancers are put into categories called "stages" based on specific criteria. Stage I cancers are usually small and have not spread outside of where they started. Stage IV tumors are large and have spread outside of the original location. Most early-stage (I and II) cancers of the head and neck are curable. Advanced-stage (III and IV) cancers are more difficult to treat, but may also be controlled with today's aggressive treatments.

15. Is cancer contagious?

No, cancer is not contagious. Cancers can not be caught by being close to or touching someone who has cancer.

16. Who gets cancer?

More than one million people in the United States get cancer each year. Nearly half of all American men and more than one-third of American women will have some type of cancer at some point during their lifetime. Anyone can get cancer at any age. About three-quarters of all cancers occur in people over the age of 55. Cancer can affect people of all racial and ethnic groups.

Today, nearly ten million people are living with cancer or have been cured of the disease. The sooner a cancer is found and the sooner treatment begins, the better a patient's chances are of a cure. That is why early detection of cancer is such an important weapon in the fight against cancer.

17. Did I cause my cancer?

No, you did not cause your cancer. All the factors that lead to cancer are still being discovered. Things that can make cancer more likely to occur are called **risk factors**, and include things controllable and uncontrollable. Avoiding certain risky behaviors (like smoking) decreases the chances of contracting cancer, especially of the head and neck, esophagus, and lungs, but not everyone who smokes gets cancer.

Risk Factors

anything that increases a person's chance of developing a disease

18. What are risk factors?

A risk factor is anything that increases a person's chance of developing a disease. There are internal and external risk factors. Internal risk factors cannot be changed and external risk factors can. Internal risk factors are inherited genes or traits such as a person's age, sex, and family medical history. External risk factors are things such as the environment (exposure to chemicals) or lifestyle (smoking, drinking alcohol). We can modify our behavior or environment to help minimize our risk of developing disease.

A person who has a risk factor for cancer is more likely to develop the disease at some point in their lives. However, having one or more risk factors does not mean that a person will get cancer. Some people may have more than one risk factor for head and neck cancer and never develop the disease, while others who do develop cancer have no apparent risk factors. Even when a person who has a risk factor is diagnosed with head and neck cancer, there is no way to prove that the risk factor actually caused the cancer.

PART TWO

Risk and Prevention

What are the risk factors for developing cancer of the
head and neck?

If someone in my family has head and neck cancer,
how does that affect my risk?

What can I do to prevent head and neck cancer?
Have medications or vitamins been proven to
decrease the risk?

More . . .

19. What are the risk factors for developing cancer of the head and neck?

Identifying the various factors that place an individual at risk for head and neck cancer is the first step toward preventing the disease. Here are some of the known risk factors:

Individual or Lifestyle Factors

Age: Head and neck cancer occurs most often in people over the age of 55.

Gender: Men are four times more likely than women to get head and neck cancer; however, this is changing. The number of women who began smoking after World War II increased, and now, 40-plus years later, more women are being diagnosed with head and neck cancer.

Race: Cancer of the lip occurs predominantly in white men and is more likely to develop in people with light-colored skin who have been in the sun a lot. Nasopharynx cancers are endemic in parts of China (especially the Guangdong region of China), and Chinese-Americans born in the United States have an increased risk of developing nasopharynx cancer.

p53 and EGFR: Molecular markers evaluated from tumor specimens may indicate the level of aggressiveness of a particular patient's head and neck tumor. For example, the presence of p53 gene mutation, or the over-expression of the Epidermal Growth Factor Receptor (EGFR), indicates increased tumor aggressiveness, while the presence of the Human Papilloma Virus (HPV) in oral cavity and oropharynx tumors usually indicates a better prognosis.

Tobacco Use: Smoking cigarettes, cigars or pipes, chewing tobacco, or dipping snuff accounts for 80–90% of cancers of the head and neck and one-third of all cancer deaths. A number of studies have shown that cigar and pipe smokers have the same risk as cigarette smokers. Studies indicate that smokeless chewing tobacco users are at particular risk for developing oral cancer. Pipe smokers are especially prone to cancer of the lip. The risk is much greater for longtime users, making the use of snuff or chewing tobacco among young people a special concern.

People who stop smoking can greatly decrease their risk of head and neck cancer. The risk of developing other cancers such as cancer of the lung, mouth, pancreas, bladder, and esophagus is also decreased when smoking is stopped. Also, quitting smoking reduces the chance that someone who has already had head and neck cancer will get a second cancer of the head and neck area.

People who stop smoking can greatly decrease their risk of head and neck cancer.

Special counseling or self-help groups may be useful for those who are trying to give up tobacco. Some hospitals have groups for people who want to quit. The Cancer Information Service and the American Cancer Society may also have information about groups in local areas to help with quitting.

Alcohol Use: People who drink alcohol are more likely to develop head and neck cancer than people who do not drink. The risk increases with the amount of alcohol that is consumed. The risk increases more if the person drinks alcohol and also smokes tobacco. Scientists believe that these substances increase each other's harmful effects.

Some studies have shown that many people who develop oral cancer have a history of **leukoplakia,** a whitish patch inside the mouth. The causes of leukoplakia are not well understood, but it is commonly associated with heavy use of tobacco and alcohol. The condition occurs in irritated areas, such as the gums and mouth lining of smokeless tobacco users and the lower lip of pipe smokers.

Leukoplakia
a whitish patch inside the mouth

Another condition, **erythroplakia,** appears as a red patch in the mouth. Erythroplakia occurs most often in people 60–70 years of age. Early diagnosis and treatment of leukoplakia and

Erythroplakia
appears as a red patch in the mouth

erythroplakia are important because cancer may develop in these patchy areas.

Diet: Some studies suggest that having certain viruses or a diet low in vitamin A may increase the chance of getting head and neck cancer. Other studies suggest that "richly colored" foods (carrots, squash, greens) may decrease risk of recurrence. Nasopharynx cancer has been found to be associated with eating salted, smoked fish. In general, a well-balanced diet is recommended.

Occupation: Workers exposed to sulfuric acid mist or nickel have an increased risk of head and neck cancer. Also, working with asbestos can increase the risk of this disease. Asbestos workers should follow work and safety rules to avoid inhaling asbestos fibers. Additionally, exposure to dry cleaning solvents, auto body shop paints, and formaldehyde may increase risk of developing head and neck cancer.

Sun Exposure: Cancer of the skin can be caused by excessive exposure to the sun and is common in farmers and sailors. This risk can be avoided with the use of a lotion and lip balm containing a sunscreen with an SPF of at least 30. Wearing a hat with a brim can also block the sun's harmful rays.

Medical Conditions: Human Papilloma Virus has been implicated in tonsil cancers, and active Epstein Barr Virus infection is associated with nasopharyngeal carcinoma.

Personal History of Head and Neck Cancer: Almost one in four people who have had head and neck cancer will develop a second primary head and neck cancer.

Gastroesophageal Reflux Disease (GERD): This disease causes stomach acid to flow up the esophagus to the underside of the larynx. This condition irritates the voice box, which then increases a person's risk for developing cancer of the larynx.

Gastroesophageal Reflux Disease (GERD)

a condition that causes stomach acid to flow up the esophagus to the underside of the larynx

Most people who have these risk factors do not get head and neck cancer. If you are concerned about your chance of getting a cancer of the head and neck area, you should discuss this concern with your health care provider. Your health care provider may suggest ways to reduce your risk and can plan an appropriate schedule for checkups.

A growing number of younger people (especially younger women) with no known risk factors are being diagnosed with this disease. In many cases, the cause remains unknown. So just because you don't fit the "high-risk profile" for head and neck cancer, doesn't mean that you don't need to worry about getting it.

- Valerie Goldstein, patient

20. If someone in my family has head and neck cancer, how does that affect my risk?

Cancer cells develop because of damage to **DNA**. This substance is in every cell and directs all of its activities. Most of the time when DNA becomes damaged, the body is able to repair it. In cancer cells, the damaged DNA is not repaired. People can inherit damaged DNA, which accounts for inherited cancers. Often, though, a person's DNA becomes damaged by exposure to something in the environment, like smoking.

Deoxyribonucleic Acid (DNA)

a substance found in every cell, which directs all of the cell's activities

It has been estimated that up to 10% of all cancers have a strong hereditary component. Several studies have suggested a threefold higher risk of developing an oropharyngeal cancer in populations that have a first-degree relative with head and neck cancer.

Cancer cannot be passed on from parent to child the same way that height and eye color are. While some cancers do have genetic risk factors, most people with cancer have not inherited the disease, nor do they pass it on to their children.

Cancer cannot be passed on from parent to child the same way that height and eye color are..

People whose close blood relatives (parents or siblings) have certain types of cancer may be at increased risk for those cancers. A person's risk for developing cancer is also strongly influenced by environment and lifestyle factors such as diet, hormone changes, and exposure to cancer-causing substances.

21. What can I do to prevent head and neck cancer? Have medications or vitamins been proven to decrease the risk?

Retinoids

comprise natural and synthetic derivatives of vitamin A that help regulate many essential biologic functions

Decades of scientific studies and initial clinical trials have indicated a potential role for the classical **retinoids** in cancer chemoprevention. The concept of clinical cancer chemoprevention is based largely on preclinical and early clinical studies in which retinoids suppressed epithelial carcinogenesis. Retinoids comprise natural and synthetic derivatives of vitamin A that help regulate many essential biologic functions.

Isotretinoin

is a synthetic vitamin A derivative, or retinoid, that is widely used in the treatment of cystic acnes

Isotretinion (13-cis-retinoic acid) is a synthetic vitamin A derivative, or retinoid, which is widely used in the treatment of cystic acne. Preclinical and clinical studies of high-dose **isotretinoin** in patients with head and neck squamous cell cancer have produced encouraging results. The dosages of isotretinoin used in trials ranges from 30mg/day to 100mg/day. Ongoing trials are testing higher doses of isotretinoin as part of combination therapeutic methods with head and neck cancer.

22. If I have already had head and neck cancer, is there still a chance I can develop another cancer?

Even if you have already had head and neck cancer, there is still a chance you can develop another cancer. Almost one in four people who have had head and neck cancer will develop a second primary head and neck cancer. Making some lifestyle changes (quitting smoking, stopping drinking) may reduce this risk.

PART THREE

Screening and Diagnosis

How do I know if I have a cancer of the head and neck? Is there a way for me to be screened?

If my nose and sinuses remain congested despite medicines, should I be worried?

Is bleeding from the nose every day normal?

More . . .

23. How do I know if I have a cancer of the head and neck? Is there a way for me to be screened?

Most people with cancers of the head and neck don't know they have a cancer. Instead, they see their doctor because they've noticed a swelling in the neck, hoarseness, nasal congestion, ear pain, or other symptoms. Though these can be symptoms of a normal cold or upper respiratory infection, they could indicate something more serious. Symptoms that don't go away should always be evaluated further to rule out cancer.

A thorough examination of the lips, floor of mouth, tongue, gums, roof of the mouth, and throat should be done at least annually by your dentist. Your ears, eyes, nose, throat and neck should be examined by your doctor as part of your routine annual physical.

Some doctors, dentists, and other health professionals still mistakenly believe that smokers and men over age 55 are the only ones at risk for head and neck cancer. Because of this, they may not look for—or may dismiss—signs of the disease during an exam, or may not do a biopsy. Insist on a biopsy if you have a suspicious lesion—even if it means getting a second opinion.

- Valerie Goldstein, patient

Your ears, eyes, nose, throat and neck should be examined by your doctor as part of your routine annual physical.

24. If my nose and sinuses remain congested despite medicines, should I be worried?

Nasal congestion is common, and usually caused by colds and upper respiratory infections. Sometimes nasal sinuses become filled with secretions and may take a long time to clear. Rarely, prolonged nasal congestion may indicate something more ominous and it should be evaluated thoroughly by an experienced **otolaryngologist** (ear, nose, and throat specialist).

Otolaryngologist
ear, nose, and throat specialist doctor

25. Is bleeding from the nose every day normal?

Bleeding from the nose daily is not normal. It indicates a problem. It may be that the air is too dry, and the lining of the nose has become friable. This may occur while traveling by airplane or living in a dry climate. Bleeding may indicate a problem with blood clotting. This can be quite serious, but it is not cancer-related. Bleeding from the nose may also be a symptom of a cancer within the nasopharynx. A thorough history and physical examination, including blood work, will determine the cause of the bleeding.

26. The skin of my face feels numb on one side. Is this normal?

No, numbness and tingling of the face is never normal, though it may not be cancer-related. It may indicate an abnormality of the seventh cranial nerve called **Bell's palsy**, usually caused by a viral infection. It may indicate some other nervous abnormality. Or, it may indicate a tumor pressing on the cranial nerve causing the numbness. Evaluation by an experienced doctor is needed.

Bell's Palsy
may indicate an abnormality of the seventh cranial nerve, usually caused by a viral infection

27. My tongue doesn't move as well as it used to. Should I be worried?

Abnormal tongue movement or the inability to move the tongue normally is a common symptom of tongue cancer. Examination is crucial to getting an accurate diagnosis and should be done by an experienced otolaryngologist or head and neck surgeon.

28. When I swallow I often have food that seems to get stuck. Should I be worried?

Tumors of the mouth, throat, and tongue can all cause a sensation of food being stuck. Cancers of the esophagus (feeding tube that goes from the throat to the stomach) also cause this sensation. But there are other, noncancerous causes of swallowing difficulty. An experienced practitioner can sort this out with a thorough history and full examination, which may include **endoscopy** (using a scope to visualize the area).

29. My voice is hoarse. Should I be worried?

Hoarseness can occur whenever the vocal cords are swollen, injured, or even tired. It is common to be hoarse after yelling at a sports event, singing for long periods of time, and when there is a throat infection. Hoarseness can also signal more serious vocal cord damage, including cancer. Prolonged hoarseness that does not get better should always be thoroughly evaluated.

30. I have a lump in my neck but it doesn't hurt. My doctor tells me that I need an FNA biopsy of this lump. What is this and why is it done?

Actually, most neck lumps are painful, as they are associated with upper respiratory infections. When a mass in the neck is painless and does not get smaller with time, it may contain cancer and should be properly evaluated.

A fine needle aspiration (FNA) is the insertion of a small bore needle (a needle with a small diameter) into a tumor and then the removal (aspiration) of cells. This is usually done by a pathologist or a surgeon. The cells removed are squirted onto a glass slide and a pathologist (a doctor specializing in identifying cells and tissues) looks at them under a microscope. The pathologist identifies the cells as either benign or malignant, identifies where the cells came from originally, and determines the aggressiveness of the cells. This information is used by the oncologists (doctors specializing in cancer) to plan treatment.

Endoscopy
examination with a scope to view the nasopharynx, hypopharynx, and oropharynx

Prolonged hoarseness that does not get better should always be thoroughly evaluated.

31. My doctor says I need a CAT scan and a PET scan to evaluate my "extent of disease." What does this mean? Why are these tests used?

Many tests may be needed to help your doctor learn more about your cancer. This information will tell your doctor where the cancer is located, how extensive it is, if it has spread to surrounding tissues or lymph nodes, and whether it has spread to organs outside of the head and neck. Identifying the extent of disease is important in planning how best to treat the cancer.

A CAT (or computed axial tomography) scan is commonly used to evaluate the anatomical regions of the head and neck and to locate abnormalities that may be cancerous. It is painless x-rays, focused on the body, that are displayed in a series of cross-sectional "slices." Multiple pictures or slices are displayed to show your doctor any abnormal masses and the size and location of the mass.

As described in *100 Questions & Answers about Esophageal Cancer*, by Ginex, Bains, Hanson, and Frazzitta, an example often used to illustrate the type of images of a CAT scan is that of a loaf of bread. Imaging the body as a loaf of bread and you are looking at one end of the loaf. As each slice of bread is removed, you can see the entire surface of the next slice. Similarly, CAT scan images give physicians multiple pictures of your body, which help to define normal and abnormal structures.

Contrast media (a type of temporary dye) may be used to highlight blood vessels and other structures. If needed, it will be given to you intravenously. Other than the needle prick as the IV is inserted, you will feel no pain, but you may feel a rush of warmth from the contrast as it is injected. Again, this is temporary.

Identifying the extent of disease is important in planning how best to treat the cancer.

A PET scan shows the functional status of your body, by evaluating cell metabolism. It images areas of the body in which high rates of glucose metabolism exist. Head and neck tumors tend to use glucose at faster rates than other normal tissues of the head and neck. You will be asked to limit your intake of food and liquids (except water) as well as refrain from strenuous physical activity in the hours before the test. You'll again receive a dye-like material intravenously. This time the injection will contain glucose (sugar) that is used by all cells in the body for energy. After the injection, a scanner displays how different parts of your body use glucose. Cancer cells are usually much more active in using glucose than normal cells, and so cancerous tissue will "light up" on the scan more strongly than normal tissues. A strongly positive PET scan is suspicious for tumor involvement but may also indicate an inflammatory or infectious process unrelated to tumor.

Another diagnostic test that may be ordered is a magnetic resonance imaging or MRI scan. This scan, like the CAT scan, looks at the anatomy of the head and neck and is useful for imaging soft tissue, especially near the skull base.

If you are allergic to CAT scan dye, your doctor may order a magnetic resonance imaging (MRI) exam instead. This painless exam involves lying in a tube-like machine while it produces images of your tissue and blood vessels. A technologist may give you an injection of Gadolinium to make the images clearer. Some people feel claustrophobic when they first enter the machine, but this usually goes away quickly.

- Valerie Goldstein, patient

PART FOUR

Treatment

What are the most common cancers of the head and neck?

How does head and neck cancer spread?

How do I decide between surgical or nonsurgical treatment? Which cancers are best treated with surgery?

More . . .

32. What are the most common cancers of the head and neck?

The most common non-skin head and neck cancers are those of the oropharynx (tonsil, soft palate, and tongue base), oral cavity (oral tongue, floor of mouth, cheek, and palate), larynx (voice box), and hypopharynx (behind voice box and above the esophagus). Other areas that can be involved include the nasopharynx (behind the nose), thyroid gland, parotid glands, sinuses, ear canal, eye, nose, and skull base. The most common type of cancer is squamous cell carcinoma; however, a number of rare types can occur, including lymphoma, plasma cell tumors, sarcomas, melanomas, spread of renal cell carcinomas, nerve sheath tumors, and bone and cartilage tumors.

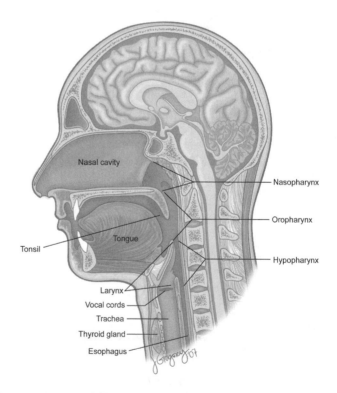

Figure 2   Courtesy of Jill Gregory, Medical Illustrator, Beth Israel Medical Center, New York, NY

33. How does head and neck cancer spread?

Head and neck squamous cell cancers can grow to be very large in areas in which they originate and can invade nearby normal structures such as bone, nerves, and blood vessels. They can also spread through lymph fluid, which drains the tissues of the head and face and drains into the lymph nodes of the neck. When very advanced, cancer cells can travel from the primary or main tumor in the head and neck, move through the blood, and spread to the rest of the body, usually depositing in the lungs. The chance of spread outside of the area from which the cancer originates depends on the location where it started, the size of the cancer, as well as patient factors such as the general immune status of the patient. For example, cancers of the oropharynx or nasopharynx often spread to the lymph nodes, even if the cancer is small. However, small cancers of the sinuses or lip do not frequently spread to the lymph nodes.

Head and neck cancers can also spread through lymph fluid, which drains the tissues of the head and face and drains into the lymph nodes of the neck.

34. What treatment options are there for head and neck cancers?

Head and neck cancers can be treated with surgery, radiation, chemotherapy, or combinations of these. Early stage cancers are more likely to be treated with surgery or radiation therapy alone. Advanced tumors are treated with combination therapy, which may include surgery and radiation therapy, with or without chemotherapy. In general, oral cavity tumors are initially treated with surgery, but other cancers such as larynx and oropharynx cancers are often treated with non-surgical, organ preservation approaches. Metastatic head and neck cancers may be treated with chemotherapy alone.

35. How do I decide between surgical or nonsurgical treatment? Which cancers are best treated with surgery?

Many factors determine which type of treatment should be chosen. Most important are:

1. the chance that the treatment you choose will successfully control and cure the cancer,
2. how the chosen treatment affects function and cosmetic
   outcomes,
3. your health and ability to tolerate each treatment safely,
   and
4. your preference.

Surgery is considered preferable for certain head and neck
cancers, such as cancers of the oral cavity, parotid and thyroid
cancer, bulky larynx or hypopharynx cancers that have spread
outside of the thyroid cartilage, as well as melanomas of the
skin or mucosa, because of a greater ability to obtain cancer
control. Early stage lesions are more easily removed surgically
than advanced tumors.

36. Why are cancers of the oral cavity usually treated with surgery?

Cancers of the oral cavity involving the oral tongue, floor of
mouth, cheek, gums, and hard palate (roof the mouth) are
often treated with primary surgical removal whether they are
early stage or advanced stage. Early tumors can be adequately
treated with surgery alone with good functional outcomes and
high cure rates. Usually the surgery involves removal of the
primary tumor and a neck surgery called a **neck dissection**,
which removes some of the lymph nodes. Reconstruction
with skin grafts or free flaps can maintain good function and
healing. This means replacing the cancerous tissue removed
with new, healthy donated tissue.

Neck Dissection

surgery to the neck
that removes some
of the lymph nodes
to evaluate whether
tumor has spread
beyond its site of
origin

Chemotherapy

a drug treatment
that is usually
injected into a vein
either directly or
through a port

Advanced oral cavity tumors are usually better controlled
with surgery and neck dissection followed by radiation with
or without **chemotherapy** than with no surgery and only
chemotherapy and radiation. Surgery often requires removal
of bone with reconstruction and/or prosthetics. Radiation is
then added, often with chemotherapy, to kill any tumor cells
that may have been left behind after the surgery.

37. How are cancers of the larynx and oropharynx usually treated?

Small and confined cancers of the larynx and oropharynx are usually considered for radiation alone because of high rates of long-term cancer control with better functional outcomes compared to surgery alone. More comprehensive coverage of draining lymph nodes can often be obtained with radiation, especially when there is the chance that the cancer may have spread to the lymph nodes high up in the neck that are difficult to reach by surgery.

The Veterans Affairs Laryngeal Cancer Study Group conducted a groundbreaking study for large, bulky, advanced larynx cancers. This study showed that patients with advanced voice box cancers that usually would need total voice box removal could instead be treated by chemotherapy and **radiation therapy** without surgery, and have the same survival rates. In the study, if the chemotherapy and radiation therapy didn't work, about one-third of the patients went ahead with voice box removal. However, a full two-thirds of the patients in the study didn't need this surgery and both groups lived equally as long.

Quality-of-life scores were higher in patients undergoing chemotherapy and radiation, showing less depression and better swallowing than those who had the voice box removal up front. How best to treat patients is continuously studied, leading to changes in recommendations. Since the Laryngeal Cancer Study Group research was completed, another study has shown that chemotherapy given *during* radiation is superior to chemotherapy *followed by* radiation in its ability to save the voice box. Complete removal of the voice box, or total **laryngectomy**, is usually reserved to save patients who have cancer come back after chemoradiation. Up to 75% of patients who have had cancer recur after chemoradiation have been saved by having their voice box removed at that time. Finding recurrences early, before they grow too large, is very important.

Radiation Therapy
uses high-energy beams that have the ability to kill tumor cells by disrupting their ability to reproduce or exist. Radiation therapy cannot be seen, smelled, touched, or felt. Just like chest x-rays, dental x-rays, and CAT scans, radiation beams are invisible.

Laryngectomy
surgery to remove the voice box (larynx)

Finding recurrences early, before they grow too large, is very important.

For patients with more aggressive voice box cancers that invade the thyroid cartilage, total removal of the voice box is usually recommended. Chemotherapy and radiation therapy, given together, rarely cures these cancers. Quality of life after this treatment is poor because patients' ability to swallow and talk is permanently affected.

Concurrent chemoradiation (chemotherapy and radiation therapy given at the same time) is usually the treatment recommended for advanced oropharynx cancers. This is because of high cancer control rates, better preservation of function, and equal survival outcomes when compared with surgery.

38. What is the best treatment for hypopharynx cancer?

Early-stage hypopharynx cancers can be treated adequately with surgery or radiation alone. Intermediate-stage hypopharynx cancers are usually treated with chemoradiation up front while advanced-stage hypopharynx cancers that are bulky or have invaded the cricoid/thyroid cartilage are best managed with surgery, sometimes followed by radiation therapy and/or chemotherapy.

39. What is chemotherapy and does everyone get it?

Chemotherapy is a drug treatment that is usually injected into a vein either directly or through a port. The drug enters the blood circulation and potentially kills cancer cells everywhere in the body, including the location where the cancer originates. It also kills cancer cells in areas to which the cancer may have spread such as the lymph nodes, lungs, or bones. Neoadjuvant chemotherapy is the use of chemotherapy before surgery or radiation to shrink tumors. Chemotherapy used before radiation may help predict how a tumor will respond to radiation therapy.

Concurrent chemotherapy is chemotherapy *given at the same time* as the radiation. Giving the chemotherapy at this time may make the tumor more sensitive to radiation, a process called "radiosensitization." Radiosensitization increases the possibility of killing the tumor due to the additive effects of both chemotherapy and radiotherapy.

Adjuvant chemotherapy is chemotherapy given after surgery or radiation therapy to kill cells that may have been left behind after the initial treatment. Some cancers receive a combination of several of these administration techniques. For example, advanced-stage nasopharyngeal cancers are usually treated with concurrent chemotherapy and radiotherapy, followed by three cycles of adjuvant chemotherapy.

Adjuvant Chemotherapy

chemotherapy given *after* surgery or radiation therapy to kill cells which may have been left behind after the initial treatment

The most active chemotherapy agents are cisplatin, carboplatin, 5 fluorouracil, and Taxotere®. These may be given daily, weekly, or every 3–4 weeks in cycles. The type of chemotherapy recommended takes into consideration the type of radiation to be given and the patient's general health and ability to tolerate treatment.

40. Can some cancers be treated with chemotherapy alone?

Squamous cell cancers of the head and neck are rarely treated with chemotherapy alone unless the cancer has spread outside of the head and neck area and the patient is not considered curable. Chemotherapy is then given to treat the whole body with the goal of slowing spread of disease and minimizing pain and discomfort. Even in an incurable situation, radiation or surgery may still be used selectively to help control tumors that are causing discomfort to the patient. Chemotherapy alone is sometimes used for lymphomas of the head and neck, but radiation may be added to improve the chance for control and cure. Also, surgery may be performed to make a lymphoma diagnosis prior to treatment.

41. What side effects will I feel from chemotherapy?

The side effects depend on the chemotherapy agent. The most often used is cisplatin, which is often associated with nausea, vomiting, decreased blood counts, fatigue, minimal hair loss, and, rarely, changes in kidney function, ringing of the ears, and deafness. Nausea and vomiting are controlled or lessened with antinausea medications, such as prochlorpazine, ondansetron, and marinol. Taxanes such as Taxotere® and Taxol® may cause temporary balding, numbness or tingling of the hands or feet, decreased blood counts, and fatigue. Decreased red and white blood cell counts may be improved with the use of growth factors that stimulate the bone marrow to produce new blood cells. Growth factors can be given to you in a simple injection. Usually, one injection is given every week or every 2–3 weeks.

Some of the most common chemotherapy agents and their side effects are shown in Table 1.

42. Should I receive chemotherapy after surgery or radiation therapies?

For head and neck cancer, concurrent therapy is most useful, when chemotherapy is given at the same time as the radiation therapy. Chemotherapy works by making cancer cells more susceptible to radiation. New studies show that chemotherapy can improve survival when given before radiation as neoadjuvant therapy for some cancers, followed by concurrent chemoradiation. Only nasopharynx cancers are treated by chemoradiotherapy followed by additional (or adjuvant) chemotherapy.

43. What is induction chemotherapy?

Induction chemotherapy is chemotherapy given first, before any radiation or surgery. A promising new induction regimen involves using TPF. TPF is composed of three different

Induction Chemotherapy

chemotherapy given before any radiation or surgery

Table 1: Chemotherapy Agents Used for Treating Head and Neck Cancers

Chemotherapy	Sequencing with Respect to RT	Dosing	Side Effects	Prevention & Management of Side Effects
Cisplatin/Carboplatin (Platinum compounds)	Neoadjuvant (given before radiation), Concurrent (given at the same time as the radiation), or Adjuvant (given after the radiation treatment is completed) (Carboplatin is usually given concurrently and weekly, often with Taxol®)	Weekly or every 3 weeks	Nausea/vomiting	Antinausea medications, including steroids (dexmethazone) and serotonin blockers (dolasetron, gransetron, and ondansetron), aprepitant, marinol, and prochlorperazine
			Decreased blood counts	Growth factors such as erythropoietin, neupogen, and possibly blood transfusions
			Kidney damage	Hydration, avoidance of NSAIDs such as ibuprofen
			Hearing loss	Possible reduction of chemotherapy dose
			Numbness or tingling of extremities	Possible reduction of chemotherapy dose
			Electrolyte changes	Hydration, careful monitoring of input
			Allergic reaction	Steroid
			Thinning of hair	

Table 1:   cont.

Chemotherapy	Sequencing with Respect to RT	Dosing	Side Effects	Prevention & Management of Side Effects
Taxol®/Taxotere® (Taxanes)	Neoadjuvant/Concurrent	Weekly or every 3 weeks	Decreased blood counts	Growth factors such as erythropoietin, neupogen, and possibly blood transfusions
			Hair loss	Benadryl, steroids, antinausea medications per above
			Allergic reaction	
			Mild nausea or vomiting	Pain medications
			Fatigue	
			Mucositis	
			Joint pain or body aches	
			Numbness or tingling of extremities	

Treatment

Table 1: cont.

Chemotherapy	Sequencing with Respect to RT	Dosing	Side Effects	Prevention & Management of Side Effects
Fluorouracil	Neoadjuvant/Concurrent/Adjuvant	Every 3 weeks	Mucositis	Pain medications
			Mild nausea or vomiting	Antiemetics (see above)
			Diarrhea	Antidiarrheals
			Decreased blood counts	Neupogen/Erythropoietin/transfusion
			Darkening of nails/skin/veins/lining of mouth	
			Mild thinning of hair	
			Sensitivity to sunlight with watery eyes, inflammation of the eye, skin reaction upon sun exposure	Avoid prolonged sun exposure; use sunscreen with high sun protection factor (15 or greater) or protective clothing

chemotherapy agents: Taxotere®, cisplatin, and 5-Fluorouracil. TPF is given every three weeks for three or four cycles. In large studies conducted in Europe and the United States, patients who received TPF followed by radiation or chemoradiation had better survival rates and higher cure rates than patients who received just PF (cisplatin and 5-Fluorouracil). Both groups had the same radiation or chemoradiation treatment following the induction phase. The addition of Taxotere® as part of the induction thus appeared to improve survival. In general, 90% of head and neck cancers will respond to TPF. Patients with advanced-stage cancers (stages III and IV) are eligible for this approach.

In general, 90% of head and neck cancers will respond to TPF. Patients with advanced-stage cancers (stages III and IV) are eligible for this approach.

44. Will I lose my hair during chemoradiation treatment?

Radiation treatment will cause hair loss only in the radiation treatment fields—that is, in the areas where the radiation beam enters the scalp. Depending on the total dose delivered to a particular area, the hair loss may be permanent or temporary. For example, where the radiation beam enters the head, the hair is often permanently lost. Where the radiation beam exits the head, the hair usually grows back. This is because the dose of radiation to the hair at the entrance is stronger than the dose when the beam leaves the head. Also, any facial hair within the radiation beam generally will not grow back after treatment.

Chemotherapy can cause generalized hair loss (from the scalp, the eyelashes, the pubic area, armpits, and so on) that is temporary. Of the commonly used head and neck chemotherapy agents, the drug Taxotere® is most likely to cause temporary hair loss.

I was told by my oncologist that there was a good possibility with cisplatin and 5FU that I would, in fact, have partial hair loss. I was concerned, naturally, about this. I prepared myself by pur-

chasing a baseball cap of my favorite team. My hair did thin out during the treatment, but I did not feel it was noticeable enough to require wearing a hat/cap.

– John Groves, patient

45. What is a biologic therapy?

Biologic therapies are treatments that are designed to reverse specific processes involved in the development, growth, and spread of cancers. Recent and ongoing understanding of these cell processes has allowed the development of "silver bullet" treatments. These treatments attempt to reverse an important pathway in the cancerous process. Common approaches in head and neck cancer include targeting a cell receptor called the epidermal growth factor receptor (EGFR), which is over-expressed in the majority of head and neck cancer cell lines. Activation of this receptor has been shown to trigger cancer cell growth, to encourage metastasis, and to help the cancer cell to resist normal death at the end of its lifetime. Thus, in-activating this receptor may disrupt tumor growth and spread. Examples of anti-EGFR drug treatments include cetuximab (C225), iressa, and tarceva.

46. Which cancers are best treated with radiation therapy?

Certain cancers are better treated with radiation therapy because radiation has a better chance for curing them (for example, nasopharynx cancer). Radiation is also the best treatment when surgery is not possible due to the location of the cancer (cancers surrounding arteries or invading the base of the skull). In cancers where the control rate by either surgery or radiation is equal, radiation may be preferred because of its greater ability to preserve function and appearance. Such tumors include the majority of larynx cancers, oropharyngeal cancers, and selected hypopharynx cancers.

47. What is radiation therapy and when is it used?

Radiation therapy involves a high-energy beam that kills tumor cells by disrupting their ability to reproduce or exist. Radiation cannot be seen, smelled, touched or felt. Just like chest x-rays, dental x-rays, and CAT scans, radiation beams are invisible.

Radiation therapy is used as the sole or primary treatment to treat early-stage or advanced cancers. If radiation therapy is used for advanced cancers, adding chemotherapy during the treatments maximizes the chance to control tumors as well as to preserve organ function. For advanced cases undergoing surgery first, radiation therapy is often used afterward if there is a high chance that cancer cells may remain in the head and neck despite maximal surgery.

Once your radiation therapy starts, it is important that you come in for every treatment. Treatments are usually given once a day Monday through Friday for a period of six to eight weeks. On Saturday and Sunday you have some time to rest and give your body the opportunity to heal itself. Radiation therapy works best if there are no missed treatment days.

More aggressive radiation treatments can involve a patient getting two treatments per day either during the last two weeks of treatment or from the beginning to the end of treatment. If twice-a-day treatments are recommended, there is usually an interval of at least six hours between the two treatments to allow the body to repair normal tissues.

48. How is radiation delivered?

Simulation

a planning session for radiation therapy

Once your doctor decides that you need radiation therapy, you will be scheduled for a planning session (**simulation**). The simulation allows your doctor to map out the area he or she wishes to treat. Measurements and x-rays are taken. During the simulation, you will be custom-fitted with a mask. The purpose of the mask is to temporarily immobilize you. This mask is not painful. You will be able to see through it and you will be able to breathe normally. The simulation will last approximately one hour. This is the longest time you will have to remain in the mask. Several weeks after the simulation, you will start your treatment.

Each day when you come in for your radiation, you will be placed in the treatment position on the radiation table and you will be fitted with your mask. For cancer of the head and neck, you will probably be placed on your back. Radiation therapy is not painful. You do not feel the treatments as you are receiving them. It is just like getting an x-ray taken. The radiation therapy machine will move around you but it will not touch you.

Each treatment lasts only a few minutes, but you will be on the treatment table for about 10–15 minutes each day. Your radiation oncology doctor will decide how many treatments you will need, and you will have to come in for that many treatment days.

Be fitted with fluoride trays and wear them during the fitting. Be sure to line your tongue and gums with gauze where you start to get sore.

– Rob Jaffe, patient

49. What is IMRT?

With conventional radiation, the radiation is delivered usually by three fields. These beams deliver radiation of equal strength. Recent efforts to improve delivery of radiation have been made with three-dimensional (3-D) techniques and **intensity modulated radiation therapy (IMRT)** techniques. These treatments are so precise so that the radiation beam hits the tumor and spares normal tissues. This reduces toxicity dramatically. These newer techniques are used to treat complex,

Intensity Modulated Radiation Therapy (IMRT)

a type of radiation therapy in which multiple beams are used. Each beam is broken up into minibeams of different strengths so that the dose is delivered to the tumor itself and normal structures are spared irregularly shaped head and neck tumors. In IMRT, multiple beams are used. Each beam is broken up into mini-beams of different strengths so that the dose is delivered to the tumor itself and normal structures such as the salivary glands are spared. This is especially important because the salivary glands help keep the mouth moist and help protect the teeth from cavities and dental disease. The greatest benefit from IMRT has been excellent tumor control rates and sparing of the salivary glands to preserve quality of life.

50. What is the difference among photons, protons, and neutrons?

Photons are the most common type of therapeutic radiation used. They are generated by a linear accelerator or radioactive isotope and can be shaped by IMRT or conventional planning.

Proton and neutron beams are created by special machines called cyclotrons. Proton and neutron therapy is offered by a very limited number of centers that have cyclotrons. Protons allow a very narrow band of radiation to be delivered that does not penetrate very far. This limits the exposure of normal tissues to the radiation. Protons are most often used for rare tumors of the skull base called chrondrosarcomas and also used for melanomas of the eye.

Neutrons are atomic particles that destroy tumors without a strong reliance on oxygen. They are usually used for unresectable salivary gland tumors, especially adenoid cystic carcinomas, which are not especially oxygen sensitive.

Accelerated Radiation Therapy

shortens the overall treatment time which theoretically could overcome possible tumor regrowth during radiation treatment

51. What is accelerated radiation or hyperfractionated radiation therapy?

Conventional radiation is given once a day, five days a week for about six and a half or seven weeks total. **Accelerated radiation therapy** shortens the overall treatment time, which theoretically could overcome possible tumor regrowth during radiation treatment. The most successful accelerated radiation schedules decrease treatment by one week either by giving two doses of radiation each day during the last two weeks (termed "delayed concomitant boost radiation") or by giving six treatments per week (Danish technique). **Hyperfractionated radiation therapy** attempts to overcome tumor regrowth by giving two radiation treatments per day, five days a week for seven weeks. This escalates the dose delivered to the tumor without increasing long-term side effects.

Hyperfractionated Radiation Therapy

attempts to overcome tumor regrowth by giving two radiation treatments per day, five days a week, for seven weeks. This escalates the dose delivered to the tumor without increasing long-term side effects

52. What is stereotactic radiosurgery? Am I eligible for this?

Stereotactic radiosurgery is a highly specialized form of radiation therapy technique that delivers radiation precisely to a small area in the head and neck. The precision comes from rigid immobilization and very detailed imaging. A patient has a stereotactic frame placed by a neurosurgeon who screws the frame onto the skull using local anesthesia. The patient has a CAT scan with the frame in place. Radiation planning is done using the CAT results plus MRI images taken in the previous week. Typically, the tumor target is small, only up to about two inches in greatest dimension. It is often located next to a critical structure such as the spinal cord, brain, eyes, or optic pathways that need to be spared from high doses of radiation.

Stereotactic Radiosurgery

a highly specialized form of radiation therapy technique that delivers radiation precisely to a small area in the head and neck. The precision comes from rigid immobilization and very detailed imaging

Stereotactic radiosurgery is often considered for patients who have already received a course of external beam radiation but have had tumors recur in a small area. Usually, stereotactic surgery is considered for tumors that are cannot be removed surgically or still remain despite surgery (that is, some of the tumor is left behind after surgery).

53. How will I feel during radiation therapy?

Significant side effects from radiation therapy usually do not begin for two weeks and only affect areas where the radiation is pointed. Patients may notice thick mucus, dry mouth,

Significant side effects from radiation therapy usually do not begin for two weeks and only affect areas where the radiation is pointed.

changes in taste, sunburn-like skin changes, and nausea related to excess thick mucus. Near the middle or end of treatment, patients may experience sores in the mouth, difficulty swallowing, hair loss, and fatigue. Most of these side effects will disappear after treatment ends. Rarely, patients can develop a blocked saliva duct with sudden painful swelling of the parotid glands located at the angle of the jaw bones.

Do not expect significant improvement for 2–3 weeks. I found this period of time very frustrating and depressing. You will find a gradual turn at day 14 or 15. My mucositis was so thick that I wasn't able to swallow for 3–4 weeks. I walked around with a paper cup lined with tissue for spitting.

-Rob Jaffe, patient

The first few weeks, I did not feel the fatigue that I thought I would. The radiation treatment itself was quick and painless. Thick mucus developed around treatment 35 (the last week of treatment). It lasted for several weeks. My throat was sore from the swelling due to the radiation. My skin became redder and burned as the treatment came to an end. I used an ointment on it that helped significantly to keep my skin moist. Fatigue became more prevalent as treatment progressed and I was sleeping more during the day.

- John Groves, patient

Just as there may be a 3-week lag before you experience symptoms when starting radiation therapy, you may also experience a lag of several weeks after treatment ends before your symptoms become less severe. Everyone is different in how fast they heal following treatment. Some people may start to feel better within a few weeks; for others, it can take months.

- Valerie Goldstein, patient

54. Why should I avoid missing treatment (called treatment break) during radiation therapy?

Head and neck squamous cell cancers can begin to regrow quickly while patients are on radiation therapy. Therefore, you should complete radiation treatment as planned without taking any time off (treatment breaks). It has been shown that treatment breaks of greater than five days decrease the efficacy of radiation and increase the chance for tumor regrowth with resulting decreased chance of curing the cancer.

55. Why should I get a dental evaluation before radiation therapy? Why should I follow up with a dentist after radiation therapy?

Dental evaluation prior to radiation therapy is crucial to prevent dental complications after the treatment is over. Any teeth that are severely decayed and are not restorable should be removed before starting treatment. Also, dental fluoride trays will be constructed by the dentist for the upper and lower jaws. These trays will serve two purposes. They are often worn during each treatment to move the tongue and cheek away from metal work (crowns, fillings, implants) in the mouth. This minimizes the effect of radiation "scatter" on the tongue and cheek. Scatter is caused by the radiation beam hitting dental work and then bouncing back onto the tongue and cheek, which increases sores in those areas. The dental trays, filled with liquid fluoride, are also used nightly during treatment and forever. This direct application of fluoride helps prevent new dental problems.

Routine, regular follow-up with a dentist is very important. Regular cleaning will help prevent severe dental **caries** (cavities). The dryness experienced after radiation therapy puts patients at risk for more cavities and infections, especially if patients eat a lot of sweets or drink lots of juices or soda.

Caries

cavities in the teeth

56. What is osteoradionecrosis and how can I avoid it?

Osteoradionecrosis is the breakdown, damage, and disintegration of bone. For head and neck cancer patients who have received radiation therapy, injury to a jaw bone may lead to delayed or abnormal wound healing. This injury can be after a planned procedure like a dental extraction, but it can also occur spontaneously without a triggering event. Osteoradionecrosis, or ORN, most commonly affects the mandible (lower jaw bone). It occurs because radiation decreases the blood supply to the jaw bone, which then slows or impairs bone healing. ORN is usually managed conservatively with antibiotics and something called hyperbaric oxygen treatment, which provides high oxygen to the bone, helping it to heal. The best way to prevent ORN is to avoid dental extractions following radiation therapy and to maintain meticulous dental hygiene using daily fluoride supplementation. If a dental extraction is unavoidable, hyperbaric oxygen treatments should be considered before and after extraction to minimize the chance for osteoradionecrosis.

57. Why should I keep seeing my head and neck doctors after finishing my treatment? Are there preventive steps I can take to avoid cancers in the future?

The greatest risk for recurrence is during the first two years after treatment.

The greatest risk for recurrence is during the first two years after treatment. 90% of cancers that recur will do so within the first three years. Close clinical follow-up is necessary for early detection of any recurrence. A general rule of thumb is that a patient should be evaluated every month during the first year, every two months during the second year, every three months the third year, and every four to six months the fourth year and every six months to a year at five years. Annual or semiannual checkups continue for life. Periodic scans of the head and neck area and chest are usually performed. Such frequent follow-ups are important for early detection of any cancer recurrence or the development of new cancers.

Smoking cessation is the best way to prevent new cancers. The preventive benefit of vitamin A or retinoic acids and interferon is unclear, but they may have a role, as studies are trying to determine.

58. How important is nutrition during therapy? How do I avoid losing weight during radiation therapy?

Nutrition is very important for patients' well-being and to ensure optimal healing. Patients weakened by nutritional depletion may not be able to complete treatment in a timely fashion and may develop infection, fatigue, and severe weight loss, which can delay or stop treatment, thereby impacting chance of cure.

While receiving radiation you should try to increase your calories and protein intake while minimizing the calories you "burn." Fresh fruits and vegetables, though healthy foods, are difficult to swallow during radiation therapy and provide very little calories or protein. Instead, concentrate on eating more foods higher in protein and calories such as dairy, meats, fish, tofu, and yogurt. Supplement your diet with drinks high in proteins and calories, either prepared drinks such as Ensure or Boost, or homemade milkshakes.

We also added fish oils (cod liver oil) and coconut oils for added calories and nutrition.

– Rob Jaffe, patient

I cannot stress enough the importance of good nutrition. I was advised initially by my oncologist to have a PEG tube placed prior to treatment and it was the best decision I made. When my throat became too sore to swallow and I was too tired or sick to eat, I could use my feeding tube. Later on, when the food no longer tasted good, the tube supplied my nutrition so my body could keep on making the good cells to keep me healthy. It was also a godsend for taking my medications that I needed to take. I would not have been able to swallow the pills due to the swelling in my throat. I would suggest consulting with a good dietician to help you select the best combination of liquid nutritional supplements to meet your specific needs while in treatment and beyond.

- John Groves, patient

Before you start treatment, ask your health care team for a referral to a nutritionist who is experienced in working with oncology patients. A nutritionist can help you develop an easy-to-eat, high-calorie diet that you can use when it becomes difficult to eat during treatment. You may also have trouble swallowing pills during treatment. If you take medications in pill form on a regular basis, ask the doctor prescribing them if the pills are available in liquid or patch form.

- Valerie Goldstein, patient

59. What is a feeding tube? Will I need this?

A feeding tube is a plastic tube that is placed into the stomach or, less frequently, the small intestine, at the start of treatment to help maintain nutrition and hydration. It is an important help for patients who undergo chemotherapy and radiation or have surgeries that affect ability to swallow. The feeding tube is placed while you are under light sedation. There is mild discomfort at the exit site (near the belly button) for one or two days. Once the tube is in place you can use it to put nutrition (either commercial products or homemade soups or shakes) directly into the stomach. You will still be able to swallow and can take food and fluids through the mouth with the tube in place.

When you have the procedure done, make sure that the caregiver or yourself knows how to use it. Have the nurse show you, in detail, the equipment and demonstrate how it works. It is a very simple process once you are shown, but if you are just sent on your way after the tube is put in place with a bag of "stuff," it might be a little overwhelming.

- John Groves, patient

60. Are antioxidant vitamins good for me?

The use of antioxidants (Vitamins A, C, and E) during radiation may protect the tumor from radiation and is not advised. Some studies suggest that patients receiving high-dose antioxidants such as vitamin A, C, or E may tolerate radiation better but are also at increased risk for their cancers to recur.

61. Can I smoke during or after radiation treatment?

Smoking during radiation therapy impairs the effectiveness of treatment, leading to a possible decreased chance of cure and an increased chance of cancer recurrence. Smoking lowers the oxygen level of the blood circulating into the tumor. Radiation therapy requires oxygen to be maximally effective. If the blood oxygen levels are lowered in the tumor, the tumors resist the radiation and the chance for curing the tumor is decreased. Smoking also increases oral dryness and worsens oral hygiene. Smoking impairs wound healing after surgery and negatively affects the function of the heart and lungs, leading to overall weakness and possible serious complications.

62. If I am a smoker and already have a head and neck cancer, why should I stop smoking?

After radiation therapy is completed, a patient should stop smoking altogether. Smoking continually attacks the lining of the mucosa of the head and neck, esophagus, and lungs and

A patient who continues to smoke for five years after treatment will have about a 25% risk of developing another cancer in the aerodigestive tract (mouth, throat, esophagus, stomach, and lungs).

makes these areas likely to develop additional cancers. These new cancers are unrelated to the initial cancer and happen at a rate of 4–7% per year. Thus, a patient who continues to smoke for five years after treatment will have about a 25% risk of developing another cancer in the aerodigestive tract (mouth, throat, esophagus, stomach, and lungs). Quitting smoking decreases the risk for developing another cancer.

63. What can I do about my dry mouth?

Dry mouth related to radiation may take up to two years to improve, and some degree of dryness is usually permanent. Most patients drink lots of water and carry a water bottle with them throughout the day. Others use salivary substitutes, which are found over the counter in most drugstores. Using a humidifier is recommended, especially during winter months when heat dries the air, and in summer when air conditioners pull water from the air. Other remedies include acupuncture and medications that can promote saliva secretion such as pilocarpine or evoxac.

Pilocarpine Salagen tablets are another option for treating dryness of the mouth and throat caused by radiation treatment for cancer of the head and neck or in patients with Sjogren's syndrome. This medicine may help patients speak without having to sip liquids. It may also help with chewing, tasting, and swallowing. It may reduce patients' need for other oral comfort agents, such as hard candy, sugarless gum, or artificial saliva agents. It is available only with a doctor's prescription.

Amifostine

a radiation protectant that has been approved for use with some head and neck cancers. It is given to patients receiving radiation therapy to help minimize dryness of the mouth

Amifostine is a radiation protectant that has been approved for use with some head and neck cancers. It is given to patients receiving radiation therapy to help minimize dryness of the mouth. The medicine travels through the body to the salivary glands and "protects" them from the radiation beam. It is administered intravenously, daily, 15–30 minutes before each radiation treatment. Amifostine does cause side effects that can be mild or difficult. These include lowering of the blood pressure, nausea, and irritation of the skin at the injection site. Medications are given to minimize these effects.* Ask your physician if you are a candidate for amifostine.

A growing number of patients are finding at least temporary dry mouth relief through acupuncture. You may need to repeat acupuncture treatments over several weeks or months in order to see results. Make sure to choose an acupuncturist who is trained in treating dry mouth in head and neck cancer patients, and always consult your doctor before trying any complementary therapy.

– Valerie Goldstein, patient

64. Should I join a support group? How much should I involve my family?

Joining a support group is an individual decision but can help you gain knowledge about head and neck cancer treatment and receive crucial emotional support. Involving a family member or friend is often helpful to help you understand and grasp the complexity of treatment options during the decision-making period. A friend or family member involved can help you to organize appointments and to remember key information such as instructions on how to take medications to minimize side effects of treatment.

My wife arranged for family members and good friends to spend a week at a time with us. They were there to drive me to and be an added set of ears at my appointments. Her decision and the added help was key to life being as normal as possible for my children and helped us maintain our sanity through a most difficult time.

– Rob Jaffe, patient

---

*Patients should be adequately hydrated prior to infusion. Antiemetic medication is recommended prior to and in conjunction with administration.

Support groups are not for everybody, but if you, your caregiver, family, and/or friends feel anxiety over your diagnosis and/or treatment, then perhaps you might want to investigate some type of support. It could be some type of support group, information on the Internet, a good friend or relative, or a social worker from your medical group. Support groups can be wonderful sources of information and help for people facing cancer for the first time or a recurring time. When you can communicate with someone who has gone through your type of cancer, it can be an enormous source of support for a person. It should be up to each individual, though, as to whether they participate or not. Everyone finds their support in different places.

– John Groves, patient

Some organizations will match patients with survivors who have had similar diagnoses and treatments. This can be a good option if you don't feel up to joining a support group but want to speak to someone who's been where you are now. Support for People with Oral and Head and Neck Cancer (SPOHNC) offers a National Survivor Volunteer Network that matches patients who have had similar head and neck diagnoses. You can learn more about the Network at www.spohnc.org.

– Valerie Goldstein, patient

65. Can I use complementary methods during treatment?

Methods that complement standard treatment are usually very helpful. Many patients complement standard treatment with interventions such as therapeutic massage, visualization, and relaxation. Acupressure and acupuncture may be okay, but discuss these with your doctor. You should always tell your doctor if you are taking any herbs or receiving homeopathy treatments. Some of these "natural" products can cause unexpected side effects when combined with radiation

You should always tell your doctor if you are taking any herbs or receiving homeopathy treatments.

or chemotherapy. For example, some herbs alter metabolism of chemotherapy, leading to under- or overdosing. Other complementary medications and herbs change your body's ability to clot and may cause you to bleed from the radiation itself (which is not an expected or normal side effect of treatment).

66. If my tumor returns despite treatment, can I be treated again?

Sometimes a patient with recurrence after previous radiation, surgery, or chemotherapy can receive re-treatment, usually if the new tumor is localized and there is no evidence of spread outside of the head and neck area. Usually re-treatment begins with surgery when possible. Re-irradiation is very complicated and requires careful consideration and planning. It is given with chemotherapy.

67. Can I have children after chemoradiation treatment?

Cisplatin-based chemotherapy does not usually cause sterility but it could affect eggs or sperm. It is a good idea to talk this over with your medical oncologist, who may suggest that you bank your eggs or sperm before the treatment begins. Fertility is usually not affected by radiation therapy to the head and neck. The testicles or ovaries are exposed to very little radiation, if any, so your ability to have children will not be affected by the radiation.

68. Should I wear a lead apron during radiation treatment?

No. Thick lead blocking is inside the radiation machine itself. This moves to protect all of your body from radiation except for the areas the radiation is supposed to treat. A lead apron isn't useful, as it is too thin to stop the radiation beams. Luckily, it is not needed for you to be safe.

69. When will my taste return? How do I deal with thick mucus?

After completing radiation therapy, it takes several months to a year before taste fully returns. Improvement begins right away, but progress, though steady, is slow. Rinsing with salt water and/or taking medicines that thin mucus, such as guaifenesin, and drinking plenty of water are all important ways to deal with thick mucus. Some patients find relief by drinking ginger ale or papaya juice.

I supplemented with zinc for my taste buds and L-glutamine for my tissue healing and salivary glands. My taste was improved in four months and totally back in about nine months. My saliva improved in about a year and a half, at which time it was back to about 85%.

- Rob Jaffe, patient

My taste began to return within two months after the end of treatment. It was not what I would call "accurate taste." Some things did not taste like they used to. For instance, some things tasted spicy when they really weren't. My taste for fruit has never returned and I used to love fresh fruit. Within four months after treatment, my feeding tube was removed because I had my appetite back and food tasted better. My taste is slowly improving after three years, but I feel like I've hit a point that some things are just never going to taste the same. I did discover that something that tasted bad at one point may taste fine later on down the road. Don't be afraid to try something a month or so later to see if it tastes better to you.

I found I could cut the thick mucus by drinking carbonated sodas—small sips at a time. I kept boxes of tissue all over the house, as well, because I would spit out as much as I could all through the day.

- John Groves, patient

Changes in taste can last, even after treatment ends. You may find that you can taste sweet foods much better than salty foods after treatment, or dislike certain foods that you once liked because they don't taste the same. Some hot or spicy foods, alcoholic drinks, or carbonated beverages may irritate your mouth or throat. It's different for everyone, so experiment to see which foods work best for you.

- Valerie Goldstein, patient

70. What is hypothyroidism?

The thyroid gland is located in the lower neck just below the voice box. It is important for regulation of body temperature and metabolism. **Hypothyroidism** is a disease caused by insufficient production of thyroid hormones by the thyroid gland. About a third of patients who have undergone head and neck radiation therapy treatment will develop hypothyroidism after radiation treatment. Symptoms of hypothyroidism include severe fatigue, cold intolerance, swelling of the eyelids, constipation, and hair loss. It can occur several months to years after radiation treatment. Testing the blood for serum TSH (thyroid stimulating hormone) every three to six months during the first several years after completing radiation treatment is the best way to detect abnormal thyroid function.

Hypothryoidism
a disease caused by insufficient production of thyroid hormones by the thyroid gland

If you do become hypothyroid, this is easily fixed. You will begin supplementing with thyroxin hormone in a small daily pill. Taking this medicine will bring your hormone levels back up to normal.

71. Can radiation cause cancer?

Although radiation kills cancer cells, it can also damage normal tissues and, over time, transform a small percentage of normal cells into cancer cells. This "second cancer" develops in or near the previously treated radiation field, usually ten years or longer after treatment ended. The most common type of radiation-induced cancer is a sarcoma.

72. What is a neck lymph node dissection? Why should I undergo neck surgery after radiation therapy?

A neck dissection is surgery that involves removing the lymph nodes of the neck to evaluate whether a tumor has spread beyond its site of origin. A neck dissection may be performed before or after radiation therapy. It may involve removal of not only lymph nodes but also the nerve, veins, and muscle in the neck.

Large or multiple neck nodes are often treated with a combination of surgery and radiation, with or without chemotherapy, to maximize the chance of killing all the tumor in the neck. Increasingly, more centers rely on chemoradiation alone to cure cancer spread to the neck, but in this case, patients are followed very closely to be sure there is no recurrence of the tumor in the neck Most patients with a single, small lymph node are treated with radiation and chemotherapy and no neck surgery.

73. If I have my voice box removed surgically, how can I communicate?

Although the voice box is removed during a laryngectomy, patients can still communicate using an electronic voice box called an electrolarynx. A naturally generated voice can be created after a tracheal-esophageal puncture, which establishes an open connection between the breathing tube and swallowing tube, is performed surgically. Patients are taught to send air from the windpipe into the swallowing tube, a movement that creates sound and speech.

74. If my tongue is partly removed, will my speech be affected?

Removal of part of the tongue does affect speech. The effects can be minimized with speech therapy. Tongue surgeries vary.

Some remove a small part of the tongue and the hole or defect is closed up by connecting the remaining edges. Other times, so much of the tongue is removed that a patch is needed to close up the defect. Muscle from the forearm or skin from the thigh may be moved to the mouth to fill the hole left in the tongue. Again, speech therapy is needed to train the patched or reconstructed tongue to work normally or near-normally again.

75. What are skin grafts and flaps?

Defects resulting from surgical removal of tumor often require reconstructive surgery to help maintain function, protect important nerves and blood vessels, and improve appearance. A **skin graft** is skin (often harvested from the thigh) applied to cover an area of the head and neck after surgery has removed a tumor and skin covering the tumor. The new skin or graft provides a protective covering of this surgical defect.

A surgical flap is more complex. It involves transferring muscles, skin, and blood vessels to provide greater bulk, and to provide a new blood supply. A flap is usually harvested from the forearm area or wrist. Tissue, including the skin, the muscle, and some of the forearm blood supply, is transferred to the surgical area. This type of covering is often used after extensive surgery of the tongue. The flap is sewn into the mouth to line the mouth and to create new "tongue" tissue to help maintain speech and swallowing functions.

Skin Graft

a procedure in which skin (often harvested from the thigh) is applied to cover an area of the head and neck after surgery has removed a tumor and skin covering the tumor

The new skin or graft provides a protective covering of this surgical defect.

76. Why do I have swallowing problems after therapy?

Swallowing problems can develop after treatment for a number of reasons. Changes of your anatomy during surgery will change how you talk and swallow. Patients undergoing combined chemoradiation treatment are at particular risk for swallowing problems. A small percentage may become dependent on a feeding tube long term. Dry mouth, scar tissue formation that prevents normal movement of the tongue, injury to the voice box, and generalized swelling can all contribute to difficulty swallowing. Injury to the swallowing muscles leads to decreased sensation and ineffective activation of the swallowing reflex. Also, if the tumor is located in the hypopharynx or larynx, you will be at increased risk for swallowing difficulty.

I had difficulty with swallowing because of swelling from the chemoradiation, along with the soreness that the radiation caused. The swallowing reflex becomes flaccid or lazy when it is not used. This can happen when you have a feeding tube and you do not exercise the muscles in your mouth and throat (you can easily do this by chewing sugar-free gum). Lack of saliva also contributes to swallowing problems. I sometimes feel like I am going to choke when I am eating because the food gets "stuck" in the back of my throat when I am swallowing. Drinking liquids while eating helps with this. Eating foods that are moist is also helpful.

– John Groves, patient

Larger treatment centers and hospitals often have speech and swallowing therapists on staff. These professionals work with patients after treatment to help them develop new swallowing techniques and prescribe exercises to improve their speaking ability. They may also have suggestions for dealing with dry mouth. Ask your health care team for a referral.

– Valerie Goldstein

PART FIVE

Changes Cancer Brings

Why is it important to learn how to cope effectively with my diagnosis of head and neck cancer?

How do I know whether I am making the best treatment decisions regarding my newly diagnosed head and neck cancer?

When I am at home, I think of many important questions to ask my health care provider. When I do go in to see my health care team, I get nervous and distracted. How can I be more relaxed and better express myself to the medical team?

More . . .

77. Why is it important to learn how to cope effectively with my diagnosis of head and neck cancer?

A cancer diagnosis can cause enormous anxiety. People fear possible pain, loss of income, body changes, adjustments in their personal relationships, and other unwelcome changes associated with cancer. Because they have so much anxiety in their lives, people with cancer sometimes become upset, frightened, or suspicious for no apparent reason. If this happens, family and friends may need to make a special effort to be reassuring, supportive, and comforting.

During the course of your illness, you may express anger or hostility toward those around you. Though this can be upsetting to family members and friends, it may help to remember that people often displace their anger and frustration with a trying situation by projecting those feelings onto people close to them. It is difficult to express your anger to the disease itself (the real cause of your frustration and sadness), so you instead feel angry with family and friends, or whoever happens to be close at hand. These people, unfortunately, usually bear the brunt of this anger.

Sometimes, people with cancer become childlike and dependent during illness. This may be a way of letting the family know they feel helpless or weak. Though the range of daily activities may be limited by the disease, it is usually best for you to continue accepting as much responsibility as possible. Continuing to be a responsible adult gives a sense of confidence and control, while becoming completely dependent on others can make you feel more helpless and victimized.

The emotional impact of cancer may be overlooked by your health care team.

Living with cancer includes learning how to cope with the practical and emotional aspects of your diagnosis, as well as learning how to treat your cancer with surgery and/or other medical treatments. The emotional impact of cancer may be overlooked by your health care team. Developing coping skills is a challenging learning process, but when you cope more effectively, reduce your anxiety, and try to focus your energy on enhancing your quality of life, you will be able to manage your medical care effectively.

Meditation, visualization and deep breathing exercises can be excellent ways to relax when you are dealing with stress. Make a tape of soothing music and listen to it. Don't be afraid to ask those you live with for privacy when you need it.

- Valerie Goldstein, patient

78. How do I know whether I am making the best treatment decisions regarding my newly diagnosed head and neck cancer?

The number of treatment choices you have will depend on the type of head and neck cancer, the stage of the cancer, and other individual factors such as your age, health status, and personal needs. Don't be afraid to ask as many questions as you need to. Make sure you understand your options. A cancer diagnosis almost always makes people feel they must get treatment as soon as possible. You will have time to consider all the options available to you so that you will be as well informed as possible.

Cancer treatment often means that you will have more than one health care provider. You may have a team of doctors, nurses, and other people involved in your care. Although you may get information from several sources, it is a good idea to choose one provider to be the person you turn to with all of your questions. This provider may or may not be the one you see most often. Only you can choose which provider will be your main source of information.

You should feel at ease with your provider. Developing a good relationship with your provider is worth the effort. This means taking the time to ask your questions and making your concerns known. Likewise, your provider must take the time to answer your questions and listen to your concerns. If you and your provider feel the same way about sharing information, you will probably have a good relationship.

Before starting treatment, you might want a second opinion about your diagnosis and treatment plan. Some insurance companies require a second opinion; others may cover a second opinion if you or your doctor requests it. There are a number of ways to find a doctor for a second opinion:

- Your doctor may refer you or you may ask for a referral to one or more specialists.
- At cancer centers, several specialists often work together as a team. The team may include a surgeon, radiation oncologist, medical oncologist, speech pathologist, nutritionists, social worker, and psychologist. At some cancer centers, you may be able to see several specialists on the same day.

You are a vital part of your cancer care team. You should discuss which treatment choices are best for you with your team.

I felt most comfortable going to a large teaching center. All my concerns about being "just another number" were far from the reality. My treatment was individual and didn't feel at all institutionalized. I felt more comfortable knowing that my doctors treated H & N specifically and not general cases. My tests and scans were read by H & N experts and all results read and received within the same day. It also gave me the opportunity to relate to others going thru the same therapy. Being H & N specialists, my doctors knew exactly what my next day and week would feel like to me and had constant recommendations on how to minimize the side effects.

- Rob Jaffe, patient

79. When I am at home, I think of many important questions to ask my health care provider. When I do go in to see my health care team, I get nervous and distracted. How can I be more relaxed and better express myself to the medical team?

People with cancer often want to take an active part in making decisions about their medical care. It is natural to want to learn all you can about your disease and treatment choices. However, the shock and stress after a diagnosis of cancer can make it hard to remember what you want to ask your health care provider. There are several ways to ensure you remember and understand everything your provider tells you.

It is natural to want to learn all you can about your disease and treatment choices.

- Make a list of questions.
- Be honest about your symptoms and about how you are feeling.
- Take notes at the appointment.
- Ask your health care provider if you may use a tape recorder during the appointment for later review.
- Ask for clarification if you do not understand what you are being told. Sometimes, without realizing it, providers use terms their patients do not understand. If you don't understand something, ask your doctor to explain it to you.
- Ask a family member or friend to come to the appointment with you. This person can remind you of questions you want to ask and help you remember later what the doctor said. If may also be easier to have this person keep your family informed of your medical condition. This will help your family feel included without burdening you with answering too many questions. You may want their help in making decisions, so keeping them up-to-date may be in your best interest.

Everyone has a different style of communication. That is why the perfect health care provider for one person may not be a good match for another. Consider what you value in a doctor. Some people feel more comfortable with a provider who will share information in a clinical and businesslike manner. They expect their provider to be the medical expert rather than a friend. Other people want their provider to have an excellent "bedside manner." They value a provider who can address both their emotional health and medical needs. Many people whose illnesses require treatment over a long period of time prefer this kind of friendly relationship with their doctor. After you have thought about what you want as a patient, the next step is to look at how you communicate with the doctor you have chosen.

I had friends and family with me at all doctor appointments. I even took my young kids to my appointments with me from time to time so that they would be less frightened of the process, and to see that nothing was being hidden from them.

- Rob Jaffe, patient

It is important to keep a notebook and keep notes of what you think about or are concerned with. Then, when you go in to see your doctor, take it with you and go down the list that you wrote. You can also take someone with you that can take notes for you so that you can do the talking and then when you get home, you can review what was said. It is also helpful to keep a journal of how you feel each day and what is going on with you. When you visit your doctor, you can review that as well and talk about the days you felt well and the days you didn't, to look for patterns. A small, digital audio recorder is helpful for recording your questions as well as your visit with the doctor, with his or her permission. There are many inexpensive brands/types available on the market.

- John Groves, patient

80. I feel as though my life is out of control after my diagnosis of head and neck cancer. How can I regain control?

Loss of control is a common feeling for cancer patients. A cancer diagnosis presents many challenges for you and your loved ones. Most aspects of your life are going to be temporarily disrupted. At first, most people diagnosed with cancer will need some time to adjust to the news, think about what is most important in their lives, and find support from loved ones.

For many, this time is a difficult one, full of emotion—feelings such as disbelief, shock, fear, guilt, and anger are all normal. These feelings use up a lot of mental energy, which can make it hard to absorb and understand all of the medical information being given you. It will probably take some time for you to come to terms with your diagnosis and treatment plan—both physically and emotionally.

People with cancer may feel disconnected with their bodies and may be less in control of its functions. Tending to your medical care disrupts usual routines. The side effects of treatment (nausea, fatigue, pain, altered taste, dry mouth, weight loss) may affect your ability to socialize and participate in your usual activities of daily living. Try to remind yourself that many of these disruptions are temporary and will subside in time.

Asking questions about your diagnosis may help you to feel more in control. Some questions to ask might be:

- What is my diagnosis? What type of cancer do I have?
- What treatment do you recommend?
- Are there other treatment alternatives?
- What are the benefits of these treatments?
- What are the risks?
- What medicines are you giving me? What are they for?

- How should I expect to feel during treatment?
- What side effects, if any, can I expect to have?
- What can be done about the side effects?

Bring your notes with you to appointments to help you remember what you wanted to ask or tell your provider.

Bring your notes with you to appointments to help you remember what you wanted to ask or tell your provider. When you get instructions from your provider, write them down. Ask for information in writing if possible. Make sure you understand them before you leave the office. Then follow them exactly. You may also want to keep written notes on any health questions and concerns.

Some other issues you may want to discuss with your provider:

- Who else gets information about me? Should my spouse, my friends, or another provider also get information? Think about your options and tell your provider what you want.
- What issues are important to me? Will the disease or the treatment keep me from working or caring for my family? Will I have physical problems? Ask your provider if you want more information about your treatment. Ask if there is printed information you can take with you.
- If you have feelings of sadness or hopelessness that do not go away, tell your provider. You may have clinical depression, which is an illness that can occur along with the cancer. It can easily be treated.
- What is the best time to call if I have a question? Some providers have a special time to return calls. Expect your provider to call you back, but remember that a quick response may not always be possible if another patient is having a problem.
- Is there a contact person in the office who is available? Is there a different number to call in the evenings/on weekends/on holidays?

Above all, your provider should take your questions seriously. He or she should be interested in your concerns and not make you feel rushed. If your provider does not respond to you in the way you wish, bring it up at your next visit. This may be a difficult thing to do, but your relationship may suffer if you do not voice these concerns.

People cope with cancer just like people cope with many other problems in life—very differently. The ways in which cancer affects each person's body and lifestyle are unique, and every person also has a unique coping strategy. Most people find ways to continue with their work, hobbies, and social relationships.

As you work to find a way of coping that works for you, you may want to try some of the following suggestions:

- **Build your knowledge base:** Some people find that learning as much as they can about their diagnosis and treatment gives them a sense of control over what happens. You may want only small amounts of information. Don't be afraid to tell your provider how much or how little information you want or need.
- **Express your feelings:** Some people discover that giving some kind of expression to their feelings helps them maintain a positive attitude about treatment. Many people feel that expressing sadness, fear, or anger is a sign of weakness. In fact, the opposite is often true. It is more difficult to express complex, powerful emotions than it is to try to hide them. Hiding from your feelings can also make it harder to find an effective way to cope with them. There are many ways to express your feelings. You need to find one that is most comfortable for you. You might choose to talk with trusted friends or relatives, keep a private journal, or even express your feelings through painting or drawing.

- **Take care of yourself:** Take time to do something you enjoy every day. Prepare your favorite meal, spend time with an uplifting friend, watch a movie, meditate, listen to your favorite music, or whatever you find most enjoyable.
- **Exercise:** If you feel up to it, and your health care provider agrees that you're ready, start a mild exercise program such as walking, yoga, swimming, or stretching. Exercise can help you feel better about your body.
- **Reach out to others:** There will be times when finding strength is hard and the situation feels overwhelming. You may feel as if you can't do this all by yourself. If you are comfortable doing so, widen your circle of resources by reaching out to friends, family, or support organizations. These people can help you remember that you're not alone on this journey. They will be there to share your fears, hopes, and personal accomplishments, every step of the way.
- **Work to keep a positive attitude:** There is currently no research that proves a person's attitude can guarantee survival. However, keeping a sense of optimism can positively affect the overall quality of your life as you make the cancer journey. Keep in mind that having a positive attitude does not mean that you and your loved ones should never feel sad, stressed, or unsure. You need to continue to work through these feelings when they occur. Doing so will help you not feel overwhelmed by the feelings. Remember, cancer is a very complex disease, and your attitude doesn't cause or cure cancer.

Cancer is a very complex disease, and your attitude doesn't cause or cure cancer.

The American Cancer Society (1-800-ACS-2345/ *www.cancer.org*) has trained information specialists available twenty-four hours a day, seven days a week, to answer questions about cancer, link callers with resources in their communities, and give information on local events. This unique service provides needed information and support through the warmth of a live phone call. Spanish-speaking information specialists are available, and callers who speak languages other than English or Spanish can also be assisted.

If you have a computer, you can download the information from *www.cancer.org*. This user-friendly site includes a resource center with in-depth information on every major type of cancer, as well as an e-mail service to answer your cancer questions. Visitors can order Society publications, read articles on the latest cancer news, and find other helpful cancer resources in their area. The site also includes a directory of medical resources and tools for managing day-to-day tasks and keeping track of appointments. Some of the content here is available in Spanish.

Some programs available through the ACS are:

- **I Can Cope**—Here adult cancer patients and their loved ones learn ways to navigate the cancer experience while building their knowledge and coping skills. In these educational classes, doctors and other health care providers provide information, encouragement, and practical tips in a supportive environment.
- **Hope Lodge**—A homelike environment that provides free, temporary sleeping accommodations for cancer patients and their family members undergoing treatment. It makes the cancer treatment process a little easier by providing a supportive environment and lifting the financial burden of an extended stay.
- *tlc*—A magazine and catalog that supports women dealing with hair loss and other physical effects of cancer treatment. This magazine offers a wide variety of affordable products, such as wigs, hats, and prostheses, through the privacy and convenience of mail order.
- **Look Good . . . Feel Better**—This service helps women in active cancer treatment learn techniques to restore their self-image and cope with appearance-related side effects. Certified beauty professionals provide tips on makeup, skin care, nail care, and head coverings. This

program is a partnership among the American Cancer
Society; the Cosmetic, Toiletry, and Fragrance As-
sociation Foundation; and the National Cosmetology
Association.

- **Road to Recovery**—This service assists cancer patients
  and their families with transportation to and from
  treatment facilities. Volunteer drivers donate their time
  and resources to take patients to treatment appointments and return them to their homes.

*Directly involving my friends and family helped me feel more
comfortable with feeling out of control. I had to remind myself that
I was being treated by the best doctors, which in turn made me feel
more in control. I had to make myself feel okay in giving up some
control. I also allowed my caregivers to take over some control,
which made them better understand what I was going through.*

*Although I was out on disability leave, I forced myself to stay con-
nected to my work. I went out for walks, even if it was just to the
end of the driveway for the mail or the newspaper. I also set a goal
to turn my cancer into a positive experience in my life, although I
knew that I would need to come back to this goal at a later time.
I found my time spent with other patients to be very therapeutic.
My first day in radiation was very scary and very unsettling. I set
my focus on a patient that had a very uplifting attitude to model
myself after. I knew that I was moving in the right direction of
my goals when she told me that I was a part of what inspired her
to get through it.*

- Rob Jaffe, patient

*A support group might give you some sense of balance when you
can talk to other people who are experiencing the same thing. You
might also reach out to the social worker if your medical center
has one available. Your minister, friends, relatives, or professional
counseling are also avenues for you to explore. Sometimes, just*

talking to a friend will lead you to someone who has experienced cancer and can guide you to someone who can help.

- John Groves, patient

81. How do I talk to my family about my diagnosis?

When someone has been diagnosed with cancer, family roles and routines may change. For example, your family may need to help you with jobs you once handled on your own. Everyone should discuss what changes need to be made in the family routine. This way, you can make decisions as a team and work together to make everyone more comfortable with the new routine.

You may not be able to do all that you used to do. You may want to be independent or you may be afraid that you will become a burden to your loved ones. If there is no medical reason to do less that you did before, continue to do as much as you can. Also, you and your family should continue doing any activities you used to do together, such as playing cards, fishing, exercising, and playing sports. This is a healthy and fun way to keep working as a team.

Cancer affects the entire family, not just the person who has been diagnosed. People in your family may sometimes try to "protect" you or other family members from upsetting news or events. The wish to protect loved ones is understandable. However, doing so is not only impossible, but it also uses up energy that can be used instead to talk more openly and honestly together. If your family seems to be trying to protect you from becoming upset, you might tell them gently that their energy would be better spent being supportive of you and taking care of themselves.

Cancer affects the entire family, not just the person who has been diagnosed.

When you keep your family members informed of how you feel, both emotionally and physically, they will be able to understand your challenges, provide support, and help you make informed decisions. The more informed your family and loved ones feel, the more comfortable they will feel talking with you and providing help and support.

A cancer diagnosis often brings people closer to their loved ones. Patients often say that they feel more connected and that they love their family even more than before their diagnosis as a result of reevaluating life's priorities. For many, priorities shift in a major way after their diagnosis, allowing them to focus on spending time with their significant others and on their love for one another. It may be helpful to know that many people with cancer say that being diagnosed with cancer gave them a chance to reevaluate their lives and find strengths and abilities that they did not know they had. Some say that the experience has actually improved the quality of their lives.

This is also where it was helpful to involve my family and friends.

- Rob Jaffe, patient

82. How do I talk to my children about my diagnosis?

If there are young children in your family, you may be concerned about how they will cope with your cancer. How a child reacts to upsetting news very much depends on how the adults are handling it. While we may know this, deciding how to discuss cancer with children can be very difficult. Adults often have their own private, powerful feelings about their own or a family member's diagnosis, and they may want to protect the children from their fears, frustrations, and worries.

If children are not given an honest, open explanation of the situation, however, they are likely to draw inaccurate, equally upsetting conclusions on their own. Both adults and children can and do learn to cope with cancer and its treatments. When talking to children about cancer, you should give them simple yet accurate information that they will understand. It is best to share the information in small doses, and to keep the explanations appropriate to their age and level of understanding. Be sure to give children the opportunity to ask their questions and have them answered.

If you feel it appropriate, you may also wish to have a social worker or school psychologist speak with your child. They may know of support groups for children in your area. They can also give the child a source of support that is outside of the family's own set of fears, frustrations, and concerns.

Involving my kids in my appointments helped them understand more about what I was going through. They also understood that I would recover.

- Rob Jaffe, patient

83. How do I talk to my friends about my diagnosis?

The decision to discuss your diagnosis with friends is yours alone. It is usually best to be honest about your cancer with people close to you. Keeping it a secret can cause you more stress at a time when you could use the support of others. Remember, too, that your friends will probably learn about your cancer at some point. If and when they do, they may feel hurt and left out if you haven't told them, which may make it harder for them to be supportive.

It is usually best to be honest about your cancer with people close to you.

Before you talk to others about your illness, think through your own feelings, your reasons for telling them, and your expectations of them. People react very differently to upsetting news, so try to be prepared for a wide variety of reactions. Often, people don't know what to say, which makes them feel awkward and uncomfortable. They may feel sad and be afraid of upsetting you. They may withdraw or distance themselves.

Some may become overly considerate or intrusive. Sometimes people unknowingly react in hurtful ways because of their own fear or lack of information.

Most likely, your friends will want to help you, but they may be unsure of how to do so. Be prepared to tell them how they can help. Help may include such things as transportation to and from your appointments, buying groceries and putting them away, or babysitting.

Once people have had time to adjust to the news, don't be afraid to help them understand what's happening with you. Explain what kind of cancer you have and the treatments you'll need. Tell them that cancer is not a death sentence, nor is it contagious. Find out what they think and how they feel, and try to answer their questions. Try to be direct with others and express your needs and feelings openly. It is generally more stressful to hide emotions than to express them. Sharing with other people can be helpful both to you and to those close to you.

I received calls from friends that I hadn't spoken to in years wishing me their best. I found that the more comfortable that I was in discussing my cancer, the more comfortable they were. These calls brought all of us closer and made them feel that they were helping and involved in my recovery.

- Rob Jaffe, patient

84. Who is at higher risk to experience difficulties in coping with cancer?

Some people are able to go through the entire diagnosis and treatment and maintain a positive outlook. They manage their lives and their medical care and do so with ease. Anyone, however, may experience difficulty in coping. Having cancer is a stressful experience. Being upset and worried are part of the process. Sometimes, distress can go from a normal level to an excessive one that can interfere with your treatment and your ability to cope with the illness. It is not a character flaw to be distressed enough that it interferes with your ability to do your usual activities.

Your first line of defense in coping with distress is having a health care provider and cancer care team with whom you feel comfortable. Talk to them about how you feel. They will direct *you* to the help you need. Remember that they are treating you as a person, not just your cancer, and they depend on your input to tell them how you are feeling.

Sometimes it is difficult to talk about your distress in a clear way so that your cancer team can understand what you're going through. They may suggest that a tool be used to help measure your distress. It is similar to a thermometer or a pain scale. For assessing pain, a patient might be asked, "How is your pain right now on a scale of 0 to 10?" This has proved to be a helpful and accurate way of measuring pain. A score above 4 indicates significant pain, which tells the cancer care team to reconsider the pain medicines or refer the patient to a pain specialist.

A **Symptom Distress Thermometer** uses the same 0 to 10 scale. This assessment tool can be marked while you are waiting for treatment or an appointment. Just as with the pain scale, you are asked to circle the number from 0 to 10 (with 0 being the lowest and 10 the highest) that indicates how much distress you feel today and over the past week. Most people rate their distress accurately. If your answer is number 4 or above, you likely have a moderate to excessive degree of distress. At this range, you should be further evaluated and some action should be taken to improve your level of distress.

Symptom Distress Thermometer
no text in glossary

Not only does this tool tell your team about how you are doing emotionally, but it also opens up the opportunity during your visit to talk and work out your specific problems. Surveys done in outpatient clinics have shown that between 20% and 40% of patients have significant levels of distress. Don't feel that this is only happening to you.

Along with the distress thermometer is a problem list. Here you are asked to read through a list of problems and check possible reasons for the distress. The problems are grouped under the following categories:

- Practical problems (housing or child care)
- Family problems (dealing with children or partner)
- Emotional problems (worry and sadness)
- Spiritual or religious concerns (loss of faith)
- Physical problems (pain, diarrhea, or appetite)

A copy of the symptom distress thermometer form is included in the Appendix.

Once your cancer care team is aware that you are having problems in a particular area, they can address these concerns. A nurse usually provides the first follow-up contact after the distress thermometer and problem list are completed. She or he will ask questions after looking at the questionnaire and possibly refer you to other professionals like a social worker, nutritionist, or chaplain.

A social worker helps with the practical, family, and psychosocial issues. A mental health counselor, psychologist, psychiatrist, social worker, or nurse may be trained to help you if you are emotionally upset. A pastoral care counselor or chaplain is skilled in helping you with your spiritual concerns. You may request the clergy of your choice in many places. If your distress is mild, the team may choose to handle the problem within the existing team members or recommend a support group.

85. How do I know when my level of distress has reached a level for which I need professional help?

This can be a difficult question to answer because distress and mood swings are a normal part of having cancer. Sometimes certain signs or symptoms may be present that could be a "red flag" that distress is becoming excessive. These include:

- Feeling overwhelmed by fears to the point of panic or an overpowering sense of dread
- Feeling so sad that you feel you cannot go through with treatment
- Unusual irritability and anger
- Inability to cope with pain, fatigue, and nausea
- Poor concentration, having "fuzzy thinking," and sudden memory problems
- Having a very difficult time making any decisions
- Feeling despair and hopelessness—wondering if there is any point in going on
- Constant thoughts about cancer and/or death
- Trouble sleeping (less than 4 hours)
- Trouble eating (a noticeable decrease in appetite, or no appetite, for a period of weeks)
- Family conflicts and issues that seem impossible to resolve
- Questioning your faith and religious beliefs that once gave you comfort
- Feeling worthless and useless

Sometimes things from the past may make you or your family members more vulnerable to greater distress and need for help. These might include:

- Having a relative who died as a result of cancer
- Having a recent loss of someone close to you
- Having had depression or suicidal thoughts in the past
- Reliving a painful event from your past that seems unrelated to the current situation
- Having had thoughts of harming yourself or someone else

If any of these signs or symptoms is present, talk to your health care provider. You or your family members may need help with distress.

Sometimes certain signs or symptoms may be present that could be a "red flag" that distress is becoming excessive.

I went through about 10–14 days of insomnia at the end of my treatment. I think that 2–3 weeks after treatment ending are the most stressful. You are getting worse and you are not tied daily to your medical team. My fear of insomnia at 11 each evening was very trying. I took some Lunesta and Ativan to help sleep. After a week or so my confidence in sleeping returned.

– Rob Jaffe, patient

86. Are there any useful techniques or therapies to help me manage the stress of my diagnosis, upcoming surgery, and possible chemotherapy/radiation therapy?

Periodic mood swings and distress are normal after a diagnosis of cancer and during your cancer treatments. It is important to rely on ways of coping that have helped you solve problems and crises in the past. If it helps to talk to someone else, find someone you feel comfortable talking with about your illness. If you prefer not to talk about your illness, you may find relaxation, meditation, listening to music, or similar approaches to be helpful. Use whatever has worked for you before, but if what you are doing is not helping, find a different way to cope.

Some useful techniques may be:

- Deal with cancer "one day at a time" and try to leave worries and concerns about the future behind. The task of coping with cancer seems less overwhelming when you break it up into more manageable pieces. This also allows you to focus on getting the most out of each day in spite of your illness.
- Explore support and self-help groups. If this is not helpful to you, leave the group and explore other options.
- Find a doctor who lets you ask all the questions you need to. Make sure there is trust and mutual respect. Insist on being a partner in your treatment.

- Ask what side effects you should expect and be pre-pared for them. Anticipating problems often makes it easier to handle them if and when they occur.
- Explore spiritual and religious beliefs and practices such as prayer that may have helped you in the past. If you don't consider yourself a very religious or spiritual person, get support from any belief system that you value. Spirituality may comfort you and help you find meaning in the experience of your illness.
- Keep a notebook of all your dates for treatment, blood results, scan results, symptoms you're experiencing, side effects, list of current medications, and general medi-cal information. Information about your cancer and its treatment is important to have.
- Keep a journal if you can express yourself in this way. It can help you process the cancer journey, and you may be surprised at how helpful this can be.

Speak to someone who has been thru the same or a similar experi-ence. I spoke to one of my closest friends about my fears. She had confronted brain surgery and recurrences for about ten years. She suggested that I use visualizations, music, and motivational tapes to help me through.

- Rob Jaffe, patient

87. I have been using the suggested coping techniques, but I still feel down most of the time, and I constantly worry about my cancer despite the fact that I was diagnosed almost four weeks ago. What should I do?

Despite using appropriate coping skills, many people still find that they need further assistance and guidance. Many people go through a period of grief and mourning when they first learn they have cancer. They mourn the loss of themselves as a healthy person and the loss of certainty in their lives. This period of grieving may seem similar to clinical depression, but it is not the same. Grieving—experiencing sadness, fear, anger, or crying spells—is a normal, healthy reaction to learning of a serious health concern. It usually does not last long, and it serves as a way for people to make sense of all that has changed in their lives.

About one in four people with cancer will develop clinical depression, which can make it very difficult for a person to follow their medical treatment, make decisions about treatment, and even function from day to day. You may have clinical depression if your time of grieving:

- Seems prolonged (weeks) and appears not to be getting any better.
- Often involves overwhelming feelings of worthlessness or hopelessness.
- Frequently interferes with your day-to-day activities (such as being too sad to leave the house or get out of bed each day).

A good place to start is by talking to your health care provider if you have concerns about clinical depression. Sometimes even one conversation about feelings can make you feel better. If you still feel that you need help after this initial discussion, or if you think you are suffering from depression and/or anxiety, you may want to explore additional support options. Many resources are available for psychosocial support and counseling. A good start might be to talk with the hospital or clinic social worker. Contacting your local chapter of the American Cancer Society may also provide some guidance.

88. Should I consider using medications to help my depression and anxiety?

Medications are helpful for some people who are suffering from depression and anxiety. These conditions involve complex physiological changes in the brain and medications can often help. People are sometimes reluctant to take such medications because they are afraid that it means they are weak or unbalanced. This is not the case. These medications are meant to make the people who take them feel more comfortable and in control. Taking something to help with your depression or anxiety does not mean you are crazy.

Although these medications can be helpful, they are not for everyone. In many cases, these medications take several weeks to take effect and may produce side effects. You should discuss the risks and benefits with your health care provider. Any physician or nurse practitioner can prescribe such medicines; however, an initial consultation with a psychiatrist might be worthwhile. Many cancer centers have psychiatrists as part of their cancer supportive services program.

Many people who think they may be depressed are embarrassed to ask for help. Clinical depression is not a sign of weakness, nor is it anyone's fault. It may be helpful to know that clinical depression can be treated with medicines, counseling, or a combination of both. Treatment for depression can help a person to feel better and to regain a sense of control and hope for the future.

89. Ever since I first suspected I had cancer, I have had many thoughts and dreams about death, including how my own death will be. Is this normal?

When someone is faced with the news that he or she has cancer, frequent thoughts about death are common. Thinking and dreaming about death is normal. It does not make it come faster nor is it bad luck. The word *cancer* can be frightening because it makes many people think about death. However, people with cancer do not always die. About 9 million people with a history of cancer are alive today in the United States, and new treatments are also always being developed. Thus, any fear you might feel when you learn about your cancer should be tempered with hope.

This means that you may have to adjust to different types of treatment at different stages of the disease. It also means family and friends have to adjust to these stages and treatments and provide you with emotional support and hope along the way.

In the United States, death is something that people often try to forget about. They deny its existence. A cancer diagnosis breaks this denial bubble and one's mortality is front and center. Some people can deal with this reality, while others cannot. Each cancer is different. Some cancers, if caught at an early stage, are simple to treat. Others are more difficult to treat. Over the past few decades, doctors and scientists have made a lot of progress in effectively treating many forms of cancer. Many people recover completely, while others live for years with their cancer well controlled. Even people who continue to live with cancer after treatment often carry on with little change in their lives. Cancer, for these people, is an ongoing illness that might be compared to diabetes. Many people with diabetes lead normal lives when they follow their treatment plans. Many cancers can be treated in a similar fashion.

90. I don't have cancer, but my closest friend (or family member) does. How can I be there for my friend and her family?

Cancer patients have a tremendous need for support from friends. Those with strong emotional support tend to have a more positive outlook toward their battle with cancer. When you call or visit, make certain your friend knows that he or she has enriched your life and continues to do so. Show that you still care for your friend despite changes in appearance or capabilities.

Notes and Telephone Calls

- Brief, frequent letters or calls are better than long, infrequent letters or calls. Include photos, kids' drawings, and cartoons.
- Ask questions.
- End the call or note with "I'll be in touch soon" and follow through with this.
- Call at set times that are convenient to the patient or set a time for him or her to call you.

Visits

- Call before visiting. Be understanding if the patient cannot see you at that time.
- Schedule an unstructured visit with the caregiver to provide emotional and physical support.
- Short visits are better than long ones. Patients might not want to talk, but they appreciate not being alone.
- Begin and end the visit with a touch, a hug, or a handshake.
- Be understanding if the family asks you to leave.
- Always refer to your next visit so the patient has something to look forward to.
- Offer to take a snack or treat to share so your visit does not impose on the caregiver.
- All time is the same to a homebound patient. A Monday morning is the same as a Saturday night. Try to visit at times other than weekends or holidays when others are more inclined to visit.
- Take your own reading, puzzles, and needlework and just be company for the patient while he or she dozes or chats.

Conversation

- Gear the conversation to the attention span of the patient so he or she does not feel overwhelmed or guilty about not being able to participate.

- Help the patient focus on whatever brings out positive feelings, such as sports, religion, travel, or politics.
- Help the patient maintain an active role in the friendship by asking advice, opinions, and questions.
- Ask the patient if he or she is having any pain or discomfort. Suggest ways to increase comfort level—e.g., extra pillows or blankets, moving the furniture.
- Give honest compliments, such as "You look rested today."
- Validate the patient's feelings. Allow him or her to be negative, withdrawn, or silent. Resist the urge to change the subject.
- Don't urge the patient to fight the disease if he or she feels it is too difficult.
- When talking to others in the room, be careful not to exclude the patient from the conversation.
- Assume that the patient can hear you even if he or she appears to be asleep or dazed.
- Refrain from offering medical advice, including your opinions on such topics as diet, vitamins, and herbal therapies.
- Avoid making the patient feel guilty by reminding him or her of past behaviors, such as smoking, that might be related to the illness.

Errands and Projects

- Get a list of tasks. Organize friends, neighbors, and coworkers to complete these tasks on a regular basis.
- Prepare lunch for the patient and caregiver one or two days a week.
- Clean the house for an hour every week.
- Care for the lawn and garden once a month.
- Babysit/pet-sit/take care of the plants.
- Buy groceries/pick up prescriptions/go to the post office.
- Do any urgent errands the patient or caregiver needs right away.

- An errand for the caregiver is an errand for the patient.
- Frequent, scheduled errands are better than fewer time-consuming ones.
- Projects should be planned in advance and started only after talking with the caregiver.

Offering Support

- Provide emotional support through your presence and your touch.
- Help the caregiver; in doing so, you help the patient. Most patients fear being a burden to their loved ones.
- Offer specific suggestions for how you can help and follow through.
- Assume your help is needed, even if the family, friends, or hired help are also providing assistance.

Gifts

- Gifts should be immediately useful.
- A gift to the caregiver is also a gift to the patient.
- Insist that a thank-you note is not needed.
- Suggestions for gifts include: soft socks, brightly colored sheets/pillowcases/towels, stamped postcards, portable phone, books on tape or CD.

All my friends and family rallied to support me both mentally and physically. They drove with me to appointments, and stayed up with me when I had insomnia. Those that could not be here found their own ways to stay connected. One of my closest friends is a radiologist. He looked over my scans and guided me every step of the way. He was not able to be here with me so he sent me funny cards at least once a week to remind me that he was with me. Cards and calls came from people that then served to forge closer relationships with those people.

– Rob Jaffe, patient

*The Web site Lotsa Helping Hands (*www.lotsahelpinghands.
com*) lets patients and their families set up an online calendar so
that friends can sign up to help with specific errands. Take your
cues from the patient and his or her caregivers as to what the patient needs. A patient who has just had surgery for head and neck
cancer may not be able to talk, so communicating with the patient
via e-mail might be more comfortable for him/her than if you call
or visit. Similarly, the patient may not be able to eat food if you
bring it, so check ahead.*

- Valerie Goldstein, patient

91. My spouse/partner was recently diagnosed with head and neck cancer and I am feeling overwhelmed. How can I "be strong" and supportive to my loved one while coping with my own reaction to this diagnosis?

It is difficult to know how best to help someone you care
about who has been diagnosed with cancer. No answer to this
question is right for everyone. You may feel afraid to ask the
person how they are doing because you are nervous you will
not know how to respond to their questions. You may be worried that if you say the wrong things you will upset and hurt
them. You may feel worried that if you talk about your own
fears and sadness, you will cause the person distress. Because
of your own feelings, you may withdraw from the situation
and emotionally distance yourself from your spouse/partner.
This can lead to feelings of abandonment when they need your
presence in their life now more than ever before.

The best way to start helping is by listening. Let the person
know that if they would like to talk about what has been
going on for them, they can. You are available to listen. At
the same time, not everyone communicates in the same way.
Some people are very verbal and open about their feelings
and concerns. Others are more private and prefer not to talk

about these things. The important thing is to let the person know you are available to listen and to let them control how the conversation goes.

You may need and want to speak with your spouse/partner about your thoughts and feelings about this experience. You may want to tell them how much you love and care about them. You may want to tell them of your own sadness or feelings of helplessness. You may want to speak about your own worries and concerns about their illness. We often leave a great deal unsaid in an attempt to protect those we love. In reality, the unsaid things are often the most important things to say.

92. Will I be able to continue working during radiation treatments and chemotherapy? Should I tell my supervisor and colleagues about my diagnosis?

If you feel productive and energized by your work or if you enjoy the experience of going to work, you should continue to work during your cancer treatment. Many people feel well during the early part of their head and neck cancer treatment. You may want to consider taking some time off near the end of your treatment or work a shorter day to allow for some rest at home. Tell your health care team about the type of work you do and get their advice. Ask them how they expect you to feel and find out what they recommend for your particular situation.

Tell your health care team about the type of work you do and get their advice.

People who continue to work often feel unsure whether to discuss their cancer treatment with their supervisors or colleagues. Some people want to talk openly about what they are going through, while others are more private and keep more to themselves. It is an individual choice and you need to determine which is the best decision for you. The Americans with Disabilities Act protects people who are disabled from being discriminated against at work. It requires employees to make reasonable accommodations as long as you perform the essential functions of your job.

93. What if I don't feel well enough to work full-time?

If you need special accommodations in the type of work you do or in the hours you work, you will need to speak with your supervisor. You may want to prepare yourself ahead of time by thinking about several issues. First, discuss how you can get the most important parts of your job done. Then determine how many hours you will be able to work while taking care of your medical needs. If your supervisor is not receptive, you may need to discuss your situation with someone from your human resources department. If you have a conflict with your supervisor, and human resources is not helpful, you may need to contact an attorney for advice.

You can contact the following resources for additional information about the Americans with Disabilities Act and how it applies to you:

United States Department of Justice
(800) 514-0301
www.usdoj.gov

United States Equal Employment Opportunity Commission
(800) 669-4000
www.eeoc.gov

If you cannot work or must change from full-time to part-time status, you will need to speak with your supervisor or someone in the human resources department. Find out about disability benefits. The Family and Medical Leave Act allows eligible employees up to a total of 12 weeks of unpaid leave during any 12-month period. For information about this, contact your human resources department or the United States Department of Labor at *www.dol.gov/esa/whd/fmla*.

94. How can I protect myself financially while being faced with expensive treatment for my head and neck cancer?

When a person is diagnosed and treated for cancer, the financial burdens placed on the family can be enormous. The patient may not be able to manage the financial issues that must be addressed; many people find it helpful if a particular family member or friend takes over this responsibility.

A careful review of your health care benefits is useful to see what services they are entitled to. Many policies are confusing, so if you are not clear on the terms of benefits, speak with someone in the human resources department where you work or contact the insurance carrier directly.

Some specific questions to ask are:

- Can I see any doctor or must I see only participating providers? How much more will I have to pay to use a doctor outside of the plan (an "out-of-network provider")?
- What deductibles apply?
- Does the plan permit me to get a second opinion?
- Is prior authorization necessary before any treatments or diagnostic tests? How is this done?
- Does the plan provide care only at certain hospitals?
- Does the plan provide home care or **hospice** care with certain agencies?
- Are prescription medications covered?

Hospice
care at the end of a person's life. Hospice care can be delivered either in an inpatient facility (hospital or nursing home) or at home

The cost of treatment varies with the type of treatment, how long it lasts, how often it is given, and whether you are treated at home, in a clinic, or in the hospital. Most health plans, including Medicare Part B, cover at least part of the cost of many treatments. In many states, Medicaid may help pay for certain treatments. Before you begin treatment, find out whether your insurance company or Medicare will pay for your care. Find out also what part of the expense, if any, will be your responsibility.

If you are in a low-income bracket or are not working, check to see if you qualify for state or local benefits such as Medicaid. If you are employed and are considering leaving your job, find out about conversion options through your current plan. Conversion options may allow you to switch from your employer's insurance plan to an individual plan with similar coverage. Many group plans have a clause for conversion to individual plans, although premiums may be considerably higher. These individual plans usually must be applied for within 30–60 days of leaving your job.

A meeting with a financial counselor or billing clerk when you will be receiving treatment might be helpful. Many cancer centers have social service support. Contact a social worker to find out what financial assistance is available. Some patients are entitled to government or charitable assistance. The American Cancer Society and Cancer Care may be able to provide financial assistance.

Prescription medications are very costly. Many pharmaceutical companies have assistance programs to provide medication at a significantly reduced cost. Resources that list pharmaceutical companies with assistance programs are:

- Cancer Care at *www.cancercare.org*; under Helping Hand Guide, select "Drug Assistance Programs"
- Pharmaceutical Research and Manufacturers of America (PhRMA) at *www.helpinghands.com*
- NeedyMeds at *www.needymeds.com* or (215) 625-9609

Transportation costs need to be also be calculated into the picture. Speak with a social worker to get information about transportation services in the region. Cancer Care and the American Cancer Society can provide information and may be able to offer some financial assistance for transportation.

Keep track of all expenses incurred as a result of the disease and treatment. Speak with an accountant before treatment starts to learn which expenses are tax deductible and what you need to keep records for. The following are costs that are tax deductible for most people:

- Medical costs not covered by insurance. These include annual deductibles, copayments (the fees that are paid up front for certain services), and co-insurance (the part of the bill the insurance company does not cover). Keep copies of all bills and claim forms.
- Expenses paid to maintain the patient's health insurance policy.
- Out-of-pocket expenses, including the cost of prescription medication and transportation to and from treatment and medical appointments. Keep mileage records and receipts for all of this.

95. What is home care and what can I expect from home care after my surgery and during other treatments?

Home care is a broad term used to describe many types of medical and/or personal care services provided in a person's home. Medical home care requires a doctor's order and usually involves some skilled nursing needs such as assessment of vital signs, pain management, and wound care.

A home health aide (personal care attendant) is someone who is qualified to provide "personal care," such as assisting someone with bathing, dressing, and getting around. The aide normally works for a home health care agency and may also help with some light housework. A home health aide is not usually covered by insurance unless it is ordered in conjunction with a skilled nursing need. A home attendant (or homemaker care) can help with shopping, cooking, cleaning, and accompanying a person to appointments. These services are usually not covered by most insurance policies.

Home care that is covered by insurance is not automatic after a discharge from an inpatient hospital stay. Most insurance companies cover only skilled nursing needs, usually requiring a registered nurse, physical therapist, occupational therapist, or someone else with medical expertise. In addition to covering these skilled needs, policies sometimes cover a limited number of home health aide hours (usually fewer than 20 hours a week).

It is important to contact your insurance carrier and ask about home care coverage. This will assist you in making arrangements early for providing for your care at home. If home care is ordered by your health care provider, the discharge planning staff (social worker or case worker) will discuss what type of service you will receive and when to expect the initial visit. Often, the initial visit is from an intake registered nurse one or two days after your discharge home. This nurse will complete an assessment to determine what type of care you need, how often visits will take place, and any equipment or supplies needed.

Keep records of the names and telephone numbers of the discharge planner and home care agency, and what numbers to call in case of an emergency. Having this information readily available can reduce stress later on.

96. Now that I have completed cancer treatment, how do I know if and when I am "cured"?

Patients who completed cancer treatment are naturally concerned about what the future holds. Sometimes they use statistics to try to figure out whether they will be cured or how long they will live. It is important to remember, however, that statistics are averaged based on large numbers of patients. They cannot be used to predict what will happen to a certain patient because no two cancer patients are alike. The health care provider who takes care of the patient knows his or her medical history and is in the best position to discuss the person's outlook (prognosis).

Patients should feel free to ask their health care provider about their chance of recovery, but not even they know for sure what will happen. When providers talk about surviving cancer, they may use the term remission rather than cure. Even though many patients with head and neck cancer recover completely and are cured of their disease, providers use this term because head and neck cancer can recur.

In a complete remission, all the signs and symptoms of the disease disappear. It is also possible for a patient to have a partial remission in which the cancer shrinks but does not disappear completely.

Remissions can last anywhere from several weeks to many years. Complete remissions may continue for years and be considered cures. If the disease returns, another remission can often occur with further treatment. A cancer that has recurred may respond to a different type of treatment, including a different medication regimen.

One excellent way to move forward once you've recovered is to volunteer. Giving back to others takes your mind off of your own concerns and can truly help other patients who are just starting treatment. Consider joining SPOHNC's National Survivor Volunteer Network, which matches you with a newly diagnosed patient who needs to hear from someone who's been there; or contact the Volunteer Department at the hospital where you were treated to see how you can be of service.

– Valerie Goldstein, patient

97. I have completed all my treatments, and my provider tells me that there is no evidence of cancer. How can I get on with my life and start feeling "normal" again?

Advances in the early diagnosis and treatment of cancer are increasing the number of people who survive the disease. This also means that there is an increasing number of patients and families who need input about putting their cancer behind them and moving forward.

If you find that you are having some difficulty moving forward, you may want to find a support group, another cancer survivor, or an oncology mental health provider (social worker, psychiatrist) to help you understand and manage these issues as you work on improving your quality of life.

Further information is available through the American Cancer Society (*www.cancer.org*/1-800-ACS-2345) and Cancer Care, Inc. (*www.cancercare.org*/212-712-8080).

The American Cancer Society has a Cancer Survivors Network. This was created by and for cancer survivors and their families. It is a virtual community where people can find hope and inspiration from others who have "been there." Services include prerecorded discussions and personal stories of people with cancer and their loved ones, discussion boards, chat rooms, private and secure e-mail, personal web pages, Expression Gallery, and more.

When you're ready, there are many ways you can help others fight cancer:

- **Volunteer:** Help out at events; reach out with support to others.
- **Advocate:** Make your voice heard on Capitol Hill and in the halls of your local or state legislature. Grassroots

advocacy opportunities include letter writing and special events.

- **Donate:** Whether you are interested in making a direct gift online or by phone, a planned contribution in your will, or a donation to support a fundraising event, you will find it simple and convenient to lend your support

98. What are health care proxies and living wills? Are they legal?

A **health care proxy** is a person whom you designate to make health care decisions for you in the event that you are unable to tell your health care provider your wishes. This can be a very important role, so it's important for you as a patient to initiate a discussion of what you would want for yourself. Only then can your providers make sure that they are abiding by your wishes. By selecting a health care proxy, your family and loved ones know that you have chosen someone to speak on your behalf regarding your health care.

Your proxy can be a family member or a close friend whom you trust to make serious decisions. This person cannot be an operator, administrator, or employee of a health care facility in which you are a resident or patient. They cannot be a physician or anyone who is already an agent for ten or more people unless that person is related to you by blood, marriage, or adoption.

You can appoint a second person as your alternate agent. The alternate will step in if the first person you name as agent is unable, unwilling, or unavailable to act for you.

A **Living Will** lets you state your wishes about medical care in the event that you develop an irreversible condition that prevents you from making your own medical decisions. The living will becomes effective if you become terminally ill, permanently unconscious, or minimally conscious due to brain damage and will never regain the ability to make decisions.

Health Care Proxy

a form in which you designate a person to make health care decisions for you in the event that you are unable to tell your health care provider your wishes

Living Will

a form which allows you state your wishes about medical care in the event that you develop an irreversible condition that prevents you from making your own medical decisions

Health Care Proxy Statement

The law requires that you sign and date your health care proxy statement in the presence of two adult witnesses. The witnesses must sign this document to confirm that you signed it willingly and free from duress. The form does not need to be notarized. The person you name as your agent or alternate agent cannot act as a witness. In addition, if you are a resident in a facility operated or licensed by the office of mental health or the office of mental retardation and developmental disabilities, there are special witnessing requirements. A sample health care proxy form is included in the Appendix.

You may revoke your health care proxy statement by notifying your agent or a health care provider orally or in writing of your revocation, or by any other act that clearly shows your intent to revoke the document. A physician who is informed of your revocation must record the revocation in your medical record and notify the agent and any medical staff responsible for your care.

Living Will

Living wills are authorized by state laws and differ state by state. For this reason, there are no specific guidelines guiding their use. You should follow the instructions and sign your living will in the presence of two adult witnesses, who should not be beneficiaries of your estate. The form does not need to be notarized. If you decide to cancel your living will, follow the same procedures outlined for revoking your health care proxy statement. A sample living will form is provided in the Appendix.

99. The doctors say that there is nothing more they can do to treat my friend's cancer and have recommended hospice. What should she do now?

Some people with advanced cancer must face death. This is frightening for the person who is sick and for those who are around them. No matter how hard it is to be near them, it is important to be there for the person at this time. The person with cancer may feel lonely even when surrounded by people. Staying close to the person, listening to him or her, and being available with a smile or gentle touch are courageous and appreciated acts.

Sometimes a person with advanced cancer naturally withdraws from life as he or she enters the dying process. The best thing you can do if this seems to be the case is to take the person's cue, simply be in the background and be available whenever the person feels the need for someone. In many communities, hospice organizations also provide expert and compassionate care for people with advanced disease.

Hospice care is care at the end of a person's life. Hospice care can be delivered either in an inpatient facility (hospital or nursing home) or at home. The goal of hospice is to provide comfort to patients, their families, and friends. Hospice is able to provide support and guidance and ensure that all physical, emotional, psychological, social, and spiritual needs are addressed. The treatment plan shifts from control or cure of the disease to comfort and palliation of symptoms and quality of life.

The goal of hospice is to provide comfort to patients, their families, and friends.

If you and your doctor decide that you do not want any more active treatment for your cancer, or if your doctor tells you that your cancer can no longer be controlled, it may be the time to pursue hospice. The ultimate goal is to provide a peaceful death when you reach the end stages of cancer.

A large number of hospice programs exist throughout the country. To be eligible for hospice, your health care provider must state that you are at the end stages of your cancer and have less than six months to live. Although it is difficult to give an actual estimate of the amount of time a person has to live, this is only an estimate. Ask your health care provider about hospice care and what programs are available in your area.

100. Where can I get more information about head and neck cancer?

Support for People with Oral and Head
and Neck Cancer (SPOHNC)
PO Box 53
Locust Valley, NY 11560
(800) 377-0928
www.spohnc.org

SPOHNC is a patient-directed, self-help organization dedicated to meeting the needs of oral and head and neck cancer patients. SPOHNC, founded in 1991 by an oral cancer survivor, addresses the broad emotional, physical, and humanistic needs of this population.

SPOHNC offers local support groups throughout the country, online and print resources for patients, a network that matches patients with others who have been there, and a newsletter with the latest head and neck cancer updates.

- Valerie Goldstein, patient

American Cancer Society
1599 Clifton Rd., NE
Atlanta, GA 30329
(800) ACS-2345
Fax: (404) 325-2217
www.cancer.org

The American Cancer Society is a voluntary organization with local units all over the country. It supports research, conducts educational programs, and offers many services to patients and their families. It provides free booklets on cancer. To obtain booklets or to learn about services and activities in local areas, call the Society's toll-free number.

Cancer Survivors Network
(800) ACS-2345
www.acscsn.org

Sponsored by the American Cancer Society, this network provides a forum for communicating with other cancer survivors; it also has a listing of resources.

Association of Cancer Online Resources
www.acor.org

A collection of cancer-related Internet sites

CancerCare, Inc.
275 Seventh Avenue
New York, NY 10001
(800) 813-HOPE
Fax: (212) 719-0263
www.cancercare.org

CancerCare is a national nonprofit organization that provides free, professional support services for anyone affected by cancer.

Cancer Fund of America
Eastern Region
2901 Breezewood Lane
Knoxville, TN 37921-1099
(865) 938-5284
Fax: (865) 938-2968
www.cfoa.org

Cancer Fund of AmericaWestern Region
2223 N. 56th Street
Knoxville, NY 37921
(408) 654-4715
www.cfoa.org

Cancer Fund of America is a nonprofit organization set up to help cancer patients, hospices, and other nonprofit health care providers by way of sending products free of charge directly to them.

Cancer Information Service (CIS)
(800) 4-CANCER
www.cancer.gov

A program of the National Cancer Institute, CIS provides a nationwide telephone service for cancer patients and their families and friends, the public, and health professionals. Cancer information specialists can answer questions in English or Spanish. They can send booklets about cancer and can also provide information from the National Cancer Institute's PDQ database. In addition, CIS staff have information about national and local resources, and can suggest ways to find support groups and other services. One toll-free number connects callers all over the country with the office that serves their area.

National Coalition for Cancer Survivorship
(877) NCCS-YES
www.canceradvocacy.org

The National Coalition for Cancer Survivorship is the oldest survivor-led cancer advocacy organization in the country and a highly respected authentic voice at the federal level, advocating for quality cancer care for all Americans and empowering cancer survivors.

OncoLink
www.oncolink.com

OncoLink was founded in 1994 by University of Pennsylvania cancer specialists with a mission to help cancer patients, families, health care professionals and the general public get accurate cancer-related information at no charge.

Cancer Source
www.cancersource.com

Provides information on symptom management. The mission of Cancer Source is to be the most comprehensive, accurate, and personalized source of cancer information and services available. They continually serve the needs of people who have cancer, those who care for them, and health care professionals by providing free, always available access to cancer information.

Cancer Treatment Centers of America
(800) 615-3055
www.cancercenter.com

CTCA is a network of cancer treatment hospitals and facilities. CTCA assembles a dedicated team of experts who provide comprehensive, personalized treatment.

National Comprehensive Cancer Network (NCCN)
(888) 909-NCCN
www.nccn.org

NCCN has guidelines for managing specific symptoms, including pain, fatigue, nausea, vomiting, and neutropenia.

Oncology Nursing Society
(866) 257-4ONS
125 Enterprise Drive
Pittsburgh, PA 15275-1214
www.cancersymptoms.com
www.ons.org

Provides information on managing fatigue, anorexia, pain, depression, neutropenia, and cognitive dysfunction.

People Living With Cancer
(703) 797-1914
www.plwc.org

Sponsored by the American Society of Clinical Oncology
(ASCO); has a section on managing side effects.

General Health
WebMD
www.webmd.com

Good general health Web site.

Mayo Clinic
www.mayoclinic.com

Good general health Web site for illnesses and medication.

Government Agencies That Provide Financial Assistance
Hill-Burton Funds
(800) 638-0742
www.hhs.gov/ocr

Federal assistance is available to those who are unable to pay,
and it is provided by the Hill-Burton Act of Congress. Public
and nonprofit hospitals, nursing homes, and other medical
facilities may provide subsidized low-cost or no cost medical
care to fulfill their community service obligation.

Social Security Administration (SSA)
Office of Public Inquiries
Windsor Park Building
6401 Security Blvd.
Baltimore, MD 21235
(800) 772-1213
www.ssa.gov

Appendix

This Appendix includes:

• Symptom Distress Thermometer Form

• Sample Health Care Proxy Form

• Sample Living Will Form

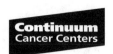

Continuum Cancer Centers of New York

Before you see your Nurse/Doctor, please complete this form. We would like to know how you are feeling and your concerns.

FIRST:
Please circle the number (0–10) that best describes how much distress you have been experiencing in the past week including today.

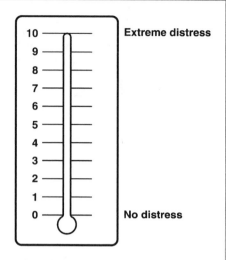

THEN: Please indicate WHICH of the following is a cause of distress. A staff member may call you to follow-up. At what telephone number would you like to be called?_____

Practical
___ Housing
___ Insurance
___ Work/school
___ Transportation
___ Child care

Family
___ Dealing with partner
___ Dealing with children

Emotional
___ Worry
___ Fears
___ Sadness
___ Depression
___ Nervousness

Spiritual/Religious
___ Relating to God
___ Loss of faith

Physical
___ Pain
___ Nausea
___ Fatigue [RN/MD: Hg:___ Hct:___]
___ Sleep
___ Getting around
___ Bathing/dressing
___ Breathing
___ Mouth sores
___ Eating
___ Indigestion
___ Constipation
___ Diarrhea
___ Changes in urination
___ Fevers
___ Skin dry/itchy
___ Nose dry/congested
___ Tingling in hands/feet
___ Feeling swollen
___ Sexual
___ Appearance

Other: _____ *DRAFT* 1/07

Sample Health Care Proxy Form

(some state forms may vary)

1. I, _____ hereby appoint

_____

(name, home address, and telephone number)

as my health care agent to make any and all health care decisions for me, except to the extent that I state otherwise. This proxy shall take effect when and if I become unable to make my own health care decisions.

2. Optional instructions: I direct my agent to make health care decisions in accord with my wishes and limitations as stated below, or as he or she otherwise knows. (Attach additional pages if necessary.)

_____

_____

_____

(Unless your agent knows your wishes about artificial nutrition and hydration [feeding tubes], your agent will not be allowed to make decisions about artificial nutrition and hydration. See instructions on reverse for samples of language you could use.)

3. Name of substitute or fill-in-agent if the person I appoint above is unable, unwilling, or unavailable to act as my health care agent.

_____

(name, home address, and telephone number)

_____

4. Unless I revoke it, this proxy shall remain in effect indefinitely, or until the date or conditions stated below. This proxy shall expire (specific date or conditions, if desired):

_____

5. Signature _____

Address _____

Date _____

Statement by Witnesses (must be 18 or older)

I declare that the person who signed this document is personally known to me and appears to be of sound mind and acting of his or her own free will. He or she signed (or asked another to sign for him or her) this document in my presence.

Witness 1 _____

Address _____

Witness 2 _____

Address _____

ILLNESS & HOSPITALIZATION

SAMPLE LIVING WILL FORM

Each of the fifty states has some law regarding the ability of patients to make decisions about their medical care before the need for treatment arises through the use of advance directives. The great majority of states allow for patients to draft living wills that set forth the type and duration of medical care that they wish to receive should they become unable to communicate those wishes on their own.

Although the law in each state will vary as to what can be included in a living will, the following sample can provide a general overview of what one may look like, and what information may be included. **Of course, before assuming that this sample will be sufficient for your purposes, you should check the law in your jurisdiction or have an attorney review your advance directives.** In some states, however, an unapproved document may have some persuasive effect.

LIVING WILL DECLARATION OF _____

To my family, doctors, hospitals, surgeons, medical care providers, and all others concerned with my care:

I, _____, being of sound mind and rational thought, willfully and voluntarily make this declaration to be followed if I become incompetent or incapacitated to the extent that I am unable to communicate my wishes, desires, and preferences on my own.

This declaration reflects my firm, informed, and settled commitment to refuse life-sustaining medical care and treatment under the circumstances that are indicated below.

This declaration and the following directions are an expression of my legal right to refuse medical care and treatment. I expect and trust the above-mentioned parties to regard themselves as legally and morally bound to act in accordance with my wishes, desires, and preferences. The above-mentioned parties should therefore be free from any legal liabilities for having followed this declaration and the directions that it contains.

DIRECTIONS

1. I direct my attending physician or primary care physician to withhold or withdraw life-sustaining medical care and treatment that is serving only to prolong the process of my dying if I should be in an incurable or irreversible mental or physical condition with no reasonable medical expectation of recovery.

2. I direct that treatment be limited to measures that are designed to keep me comfortable and to relieve pain, including any pain that might occur from the withholding or withdrawing of life-sustaining medical care or treatment.

1

3. I direct that if I am in the condition described in item 1, above, it be remembered that I specifically **do not** want the following forms of medical care and treatment:

A. _____
B. _____
C. _____
D. _____
E. _____
F. _____
G. _____
H. _____
I. _____
J. _____
K. _____

4. I direct that if I am in the condition described in item 1, above, it be remembered that I specifically **do** want the following forms of medical care and treatment:

A. _____
B. _____
C. _____
D. _____
E. _____
F. _____
G. _____
H. _____
I. _____
J. _____
K. _____

5. I direct that if I am in the condition described in item 1, above, and if I also have the condition or conditions of _____, that I receive the following medical care and treatment:

_____
_____
_____
_____
_____
_____

This Living Will Declaration expresses my firm wishes, desires, and preferences and the fact that I may have executed a form specified by the law of the State of _____ may not be used a limiting or contradicting this Living Will Declaration, which is an expression of both my common law and constitutional rights.

I make this Living Will Declaration the _____ day of _____, 20____.

_____
Declarant's Signature

_____
_____
Declarant's Address

2

WITNESS STATEMENTS

I declare that the person who signed or acknowledged this document is personally known to me, that he/she signed or acknowledged this Living Will Declaration in my presence, and that he/she appears to be of sound mind and under no duress, fraud, or undue influence.

_____
Witnesses' Signature

_____
Witnesses' Printed Name

_____
_____
_____
Witnesses' Address

I declare that the person who signed or acknowledged this document is personally known to me, that he/she signed or acknowledged this Living Will Declaration in my presence, and that he/she appears to be of sound mind and under no duress, fraud, or undue influence.

_____
Witnesses' Signature

_____
Witnesses' Printed Name

_____
_____
_____
Witnesses' Address

NOTARIZATION

STATE OF _____, COUNTY OF _____

Subscribed and sworn to before me his _____ day of _____, 20_____.

_____
Signature of Notary Public

My commission expires: _____

3

NOTES ABOUT LIVING WILL DECLARATION FORM:

- Paragraphs one and two can be tailored to suit your own desires. For example, you could redraft paragraph one to state that you would like to have life-sustaining treatments for "x" number of days or weeks and then if no progress is made and there is no reasonable hope of recovery, you would like to have the life-sustaining treatments withdrawn. As for paragraph two, if you do not wish to receive pain medications you can state those wishes there.

- Paragraph three of the Declaration allows you to list all specific types of treatment you wish not to receive. If you do not have strong feelings about any particular types of treatment, you do not need to include this paragraph in your own living will. However, if you do have strong preferences, this is the place to list them.

  Examples: Antibiotics, artificial feedings, hydration and fluids, blood transfusions, cardiac resuscitation, dialysis, intravenous lines, invasive tests, respiratory therapy, mechanical respiratory assistance, and surgery.

  Note: For many people, taking away food and water from a dying person seems especially cruel because they may feel as though the person is starving or dehydrating to death. However, you have a right to make your specific wishes known on the subject. It is advisable, however, to be particularly clear on those issues so that there is no room for your loved ones to debate. In addition, they will likely feel less burdened by guilt if they are certain they are following your specific wishes not to be artificially fed or hydrated.

- Paragraph four is the converse of paragraph three and allows you to clearly state what care and treatment you would like to receive. In addition, if you have specific instructions for other types of care, you may wish to include them in this paragraph.

  Examples: At-home or hospice care as the end approaches, feelings about religious practices or customs at a terminal stage (for instance, if you wish for a certain clergy member to be called and be present).

- Paragraph six allows you to essentially "change" your wishes should you also have another medical condition when you become incapacitated or incompetent.

  Example: For women of childbearing age, the desire to forego life-sustaining treatment may be compromised if they are pregnant. In those situations, they may wish to be kept alive, if possible, until the baby can be safely delivered at which point, if there has been no recovery or reasonable progress, they may wish to then have their life-sustaining treatments withdrawn.

4

Glossary

A

Accelerated radiation therapy: shortens the overall treatment time which theoretically could overcome possible tumor regrowth during radiation treatment.

Adjuvant chemotherapy: chemotherapy given *after* surgery or radiation therapy to kill cells which may have been left behind after the initial treatment.

Amifostine: a radiation protectant that has been approved for use with some head and neck cancers. It is given to patients receiving radiation therapy to help minimize dryness of the mouth.

Base of the tongue: the part of the tongue you can not see that extends down the throat to the voice box.

Bell's palsy: may indicate an abnormality of the seventh cranial nerve, usually caused by a viral infection.

Benign: a tumor composed of non-cancerous cells.

Biopsy: a procedure performed to obtain cells from the tumor to examine.

Buccal mucosa: cheeks.

C

Cancer: a term used to describe diseases caused by abnormal cell growth and behavior.

Caries: cavities in the teeth.

Chemotherapy: a drug treatment that is usually injected into a vein either directly or through a port.

Computerized Axial Tomography (CAT scan or CT scan): a computed axial tomography scan is often used to evaluate the anatomical regions of the head and neck and to locate abnormalities.

D

Deoxyribonucleic Acid (DNA): a substance found in every cell, which directs all of the cell's activities.

Distress thermometer: a self-assessment tool that measures your level of distress. You are asked to circle the number from 0 to 10 (with 0 being the lowest and 10 the highest) that indicates how much distress you feel today and over the past week.

E

Endoscopy: examination with a scope to view the nasopharynx, hypopharynx, and oropharynx.

Ethmoid sinus: found between the eyebrows.

Erythroplakia: appears as a red patch in the mouth.

F

Feeding tube: a plastic tube that is placed into the stomach, or less frequently, the small intestine, at the start of treatment to help maintain nutrition and hydration.

Fine Needle Aspiration (FNA): the insertion of a small bore needle (a needle with a small diameter) into a tumor and then the removal (aspiration) of cells.

Gastroesophageal Reflux Disease (GERD): a condition that causes stomach acid to flow up the esophagus to the underside of the larynx.

Gingiva: gums in the mouth.

Grade: describes the aggressiveness of the tumor cells.

H

Hard palate: the roof of the mouth

Health care proxy: a form in which you designate a person to make health care decisions for you in the event that you are unable to tell your health care provider your wishes.

Histology: where in the body the cells originate from.

Hospice: care at the end of a person's life. Hospice care can be delivered either in an inpatient facility (hospital or nursing home) or at home.

Hyperfractionated radiation therapy: attempts to overcome tumor regrowth by giving two radiation treatments per day, five days a week, for seven weeks. This escalates the dose delivered to the tumor without increasing long-term side effects.

Hypopharynx: includes the tissues of the lowest part of the throat, down to the level of the voice box (larynx).

Hypothyroidism: a disease caused by insufficient production of thyroid hormones by the thyroid gland.

I

Induction chemotherapy: chemotherapy given before any radiation or surgery.

Intensity Modulated Radiation Therapy (IMRT): a type of radiation therapy in which multiple beams are used. Each beam is broken up into mini-beams of different strengths so that the dose is delivered to the tumor itself and normal structures are spared.

Isotretinoin (13-cis-retinoic acid): is a synthetic vitamin A derivative, or retinoid, that is widely used in the treatment of cystic acne.

L

Laryngectomy: surgery to remove the voice box (larynx).

Larynx: the voice box.

Leukoplakia: a whitish patch inside the mouth.

Living will: a form which allows you state your wishes about medical care in the event that you develop an irreversible condition that prevents you from making your own medical decisions.

Lymph nodes: small, round, oval or bean-shaped structures that filter lymph fluid of unwanted materials such as bacteria and cancer cells.

M

Malignant: a tumor composed of cancer cells.

Maxillary sinuses: spaces found in the cheeks, right above the maxilla.

Metastasis: the multiplication and spreading of cancer cells to other parts of the body.

N

Nasopharynx: the area behind the nose and between the eyes.

Neck dissection: surgery to the neck that removes some of the lymph nodes to evaluate whether tumor has spread beyond its site of origin.

O

Oropharynx: contains the soft palate, the uvula, the tonsils, the base of the tongue, and the wall of the pharynx (throat) from the soft palate to above the voice box.

Osteoradionecrosis (ORN): the breakdown, damage and disintegration of bone.

Otolaryngologist: ear, nose, and throat specialist doctor.

P

Pathologist: a doctor trained to look at tumor cells under a microscope to determine whether they are benign or malignant.

Pharynx: throat.

Positron Emission Tomography (PET) scan: shows the functional status of your body, by evaluating cell metabolism. It images areas of the body where high rates of glucose metabolism exist.

Pyriform sinuses: air spaces on either side of the voice box (larynx).

R

Radiation therapy: uses high-energy beams that have the ability to kill tumor cells by disrupting their ability to reproduce or exist. Radiation therapy cannot be seen, smelled, touched, or felt. Just like chest x-rays, dental x-rays, and CAT scans, radiation beams are invisible.

Retinoids: comprise natural and synthetic derivatives of vitamin A that help regulate many essential biologic functions.

Retromolar trigone: inside angle of the jaws.

Risk factors: anything that increases a person's chance of developing a disease.

S

Simulation: a planning session for radiation therapy.

Skin graft: a procedure in which skin (often harvested from the thigh) is applied to cover an area of the head and neck after surgery has removed a tumor and skin covering the tumor.

Soft palate: the soft part of the back of the roof of the mouth.

Sphenoid sinuses: found behind the sphenoid bone.

Staging: the tests or examinations done to help determine the extent of the disease process. This also determines whether or not the tumor has spread to other parts of the body.

Stereotactic radiosurgery: a highly specialized form of radiation therapy technique that delivers radiation precisely to a small area in the head and neck. The precision comes from rigid immobilization and very detailed imaging.

T

Tonsils: soft lymphoid tissue on both sides of the throat.

Tumor: a term used to describe a mass or lump in the body.

U

Uvula: an extension of the soft palate that hangs down from the back of the roof of the mouth.

Index

Medicaid, 85, 86
Medical conditions, and head and
    neck cancer, 14
Medical home care, 87
Medicare, 85–86
Melanoma, 26
Mental health counselor, 72, 77, 90
Metastasis, definition of, 2, 109
Mortality, thoughts about, 77–78
Mourning period, after diagnosis,
    75–76
Mouth. *See also* Oral cavity
    cancer of, 19, 24, 26
    dry. *See* Dry mouth
    floor of. *See* Floor of mouth
    roof of. *See* Hard palate; Soft palate
MRI. *See* Magnetic resonance imaging
Mucositis, chemotherapy and, *32, 33*
Mucus, thick, radiation therapy and,
    39, 40, 50
Nasal cavity, *5, 24*
Nasal sinuses, *5*
    cancer of, 25
    congested, 18
    definition of, 5
    function of, 6
    location of, 5
Nasopharynx, *5, 24*
    definition of, 4, 109
    location of, 4
Nasopharynx cancer, 4, 24
    in China, 12
    diet and, 14
    Epstein-Barr virus and, 14
    spread of, 25
    symptoms of, 19
    treatment of, 29, 30, 35
National Cancer Institute, 96
National Coalition for Cancer
    Survivorship, 96

National Comprehensive Cancer
    Network (NCCN), 97
National Survivor Volunteer Network,
    48, 89
Nausea
    chemotherapy and, 30, *31, 32, 33*
    radiation therapy and, 40
Neck cancer. *See* Head and neck
    cancer
Neck dissection, 26, 52, 109
Neck lumps, biopsy of, 20
Neoadjuvant chemotherapy, 28, 30
Neutrons, 38
Nickel, and head and neck cancer, 14
Nosebleeds, 19
Numbness of face, 19
Numbness of hands or feet,
    chemotherapy and, 30, *31, 32*
Nurse, 72, 88
Nutrition. *See* Diet
Occupation, and head and neck cancer,
    14
OncoLink, 96
Oncologist, 20, 37, 49, 58
Oncology Nursing Society, 97
Ondansetron, 30
Optimism, 63, 64, 70, 78
Oral cavity, *5*
    cancer of, 12, 24, 25, 26
    function of, 6
    structures found in, 6
Oropharynx, *5, 24*
    cancer of, 12, 15, 24, 25, 27–28, 35
    definition of, 4, 109
    function of, 6
    structures found in, 6
Osteoradionecrosis (ORN), 42, 109
Otolaryngologist, 18, 19, 109
p53 gene mutation, 12
Pain scale, 71